THE RIGHT ARM

Health, Diet, and the Bible
FOR TODAY

By
Jerry P. Hasselmeier

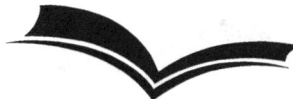

TEACH Services, Inc.
P U B L I S H I N G
www.TEACHServices.com • (800) 367-1844

Copyright © 2013 TEACH Services, Inc.
ISBN-13: 978-1-47960-034-2 (Paperback)
ISBN-13: 978-1-47960-035-9 (ePub)
ISBN-13: 978-1-47960-036-6 (Mobi)
Library of Congress Control Number: 2013950871

All scripture quotations are taken from the King James Version. Public domain.

Published by

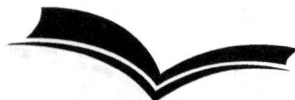

TEACH Services, Inc.
P U B L I S H I N G
www.TEACHServices.com • (800) 367-1844

Contents

Chapter One
BEGINNINGS

When God first created Adam and Eve, He formed them in perfection. Their appearance and their functions were perfect as was the environment God created for them to inhabit. They did not lack anything they needed.

The Holy Bible tells us of God's perfection and the original plan He had for us. However, as we look around the world we live in today, we see that humanity is far from perfection, and even nature has fallen from its ideal state in Eden. We face all types of problems today—crime, violence, immorality, and political and financial problems abound. We know that these problems will be swept away when Jesus returns to take the righteous home with Him, but does God have a solution while we are living on this earth today? Yes, He does. Not only is this solution for today, but it is for eternity.

"In the beginning God created the heaven and the earth" (Gen. 1:1). This is the first verse in the Bible and probably the most well-known. Jesus made reference to both that text and that period of time when He debated with the Pharisees, a powerful and highly respected sect of Judaism, regarding the subject of marriage and divorce. The Pharisees were trying to prove to Jesus that according to the laws of Moses it was lawful "for a man to put away his wife" for any reason at all (Matt. 19:3), but Jesus responded that God's ideal plan for humanity was not found in the Mosaic law. Instead, God had established the perfect plan for humanity "at the beginning" when He first created them.

Likewise the laws and ordinances given to the Jews through Moses were put in place because of their refusal to obey God. This is clearly shown in the following verses: "They say unto him, Why did Moses then command to give a writing of divorcement, and to put her away?" To which Jesus replied, "Moses because of the hardness of your hearts suffered [allowed] you to put away your wives: but from the beginning it was not so" (verses 7, 8).

So according to Jesus, how do we apply God's perfect plan in a practical way for our daily lives? It's very simple. Pick up your Bible, and turn to page one. Let me say here, though, that we should not make the mistake that some do of focusing on what the Bible does *not* tell us. What God reveals to us in Scripture is very important, and we should make the most of the light He gives us right now, not always stretching our efforts to find the unknown as Eve did. Rest assured, although there may appear to be "gaps" in Bible history from our limited perspective, God has given us every bit of knowledge we need to get us out of our huge dilemma, and a mass of unnecessary information would only hold us back.

When God first created Adam and Eve in the Garden of Eden, they were perfect in every way—physically, mentally, and spiritually. In this perfect environment, God gave our first parents a perfect diet to follow: "And God said, Behold, I have given you every herb bearing seed, which is upon the face of all the earth, and every tree, in the which is the fruit of a tree yielding seed; to you it shall be for meat [food]" (Gen. 1:29).

Thus, the original plan for our food included "every herb bearing seed," which included unripe grains, tender legumes, and the oily seeds of certain plants, as well as "the fruit of a tree yielding seed." Basically, the fruits and edible seeds of the earth were to be our fare. And for the animals, the Lord had given "every green herb for meat, and it was so" (verse 30).

The Lord also gave Adam an ideal line of work in the garden. One that would perfectly complement his lifestyle and diet: "And the Lord God took the man, and put him into the garden of Eden to dress [cultivate] it and to keep it" (Gen. 2:15). So we see that even in paradise slothful living was not to be tolerated. Keeping busy and working outdoors among the plants and the trees was part of God's original and perfect design for our lives.

Agriculture is not meant to be menial labor—it was designed by the Creator to be the work of kings and queens, princes and princesses in God's kingdom. Anyone who has a plot of land that could be devoted for the growing of trees and plants for both food and décor would benefit by pursuing this course. There is no food quite so pleasing to eat as that grown by the work of one's own hands. If all the work done today for the development of human inventions and technology were to be devoted for the development of scientific agriculturalism, the entire planet would receive a blessing thereby beyond our imaginations.

We know what God's ideal diet was in the Garden of Eden, but when and how did the human diet change? The obvious answer is the introduction of sin into the world. After Adam and Eve fell, God had to come up with a plan to bail them out of what they had gotten themselves into. We find the consequences of their sin and God's plan in the following verses: "Cursed is the ground for thy sake; in sorrow shalt thou eat of it all the days of thy life. Thorns also and thistles shall it bring forth to thee; and thou shalt eat the herb of the field; In the sweat of thy face shalt thou eat bread [food], till thou return unto the ground; for out of it wast thou taken: for dust thou art, and unto dust shalt thou return" (Gen. 3:17–19).

I would like to take note here that this bailout plan referred to here is not to be mistaken for the promise given of the coming Messiah (Gen. 3:15; Isa. 53), but it is, nonetheless, tied directly to that promise. With that in mind, we can deduce from the previously quoted texts that the "curse" given to Adam, after he fell from grace had two components. First, there was to be an increase in the difficulty of labor, and second, there was to be a change in the diet. Both of these changes were essential to humanity's survival, and mankind's long-term survival was essential for God's plan of salvation, which depended upon the coming of the Savior, Christ our King, to rescue us.

Physically, humanity needed a "life-extender" after sinning against God. Adam and Eve had willingly chosen to literally disconnect themselves from the great Power Source of all life. It would be only natural that after Adam and Eve were put out of the garden and separated from the glory of God that their own life force within them would begin to wane like that of an uncharged battery. After all, apart from God, we are all mortal beings and subject to death. It could be reasoned that every generation following Adam would be weaker than the previous one until the human race would deteriorate and die out. But, interestingly enough, this is not what happened.   Adam, with all his great might and force, lived to be 930 years. That's right! Nearly a thousand years old! But he wasn't the longest-lived of the human race. Methuselah, the oldest person recorded in Bible history, lived to be 969 years old, and he was the seventh generation after Adam! And Noah, the ninth generation after Adam, lived to the age of 950! How is that possible?

Along with hard outdoor labor, God had added to humanity's otherwise perfect diet a new element that was previously intended only for the animals in Eden. It was the "green herb" that was given to him when God told Adam "and thou shalt eat the herb of the field" (Gen. 3:18). Of this the psalmist wrote, "He causeth the grass to grow for the cattle, and herb for the service of man: that he may bring forth food out of the earth" (Ps. 104:14).

There are substances in the green herb that have incredible nutritional and health-promoting properties, things that modern science has not even come close to discovering. I speak of nothing "mystical" or "supernatural" here. This is all purely scientific, as all true science is in harmony with natural law, but because of humanity's slowness in discovering these aspects of God's amazing and wonderful creation, this in no way denigrates the power of the truths present in nature. Did chlorophyll, the substance in green leaves that allows for photosynthesis to take place, exist before it was discovered by human beings? Yes, indeed; we surely did not need to wait for scientific experts and researchers to tell us so to have the plants grow! It is simply by observing and harmoniously working with nature, in harmony with the truths revealed to us in Scripture, that we really come to an understanding of ourselves and the world around us.

Looking at the Garden of Eden, we get a glimpse of God's perfect diet for His children. Then, as we look forward to Eden restored, we also see another glimpse of God's perfect diet.

We are told by the prophet Malachi that the saints in heaven, when the Garden of Eden is restored, will "grow up as calves of the stall" (Mal. 4:2; compare to Gen. 1:30; 3:18; and Dan. 4). And correspondingly, in the book of Revelation John tells us that the saints will eat the fruits of the tree of life and that "the leaves of the tree were for the healing of the nations" (Rev. 22:2). Thus we see that in heaven, as the saints of God are regenerating from the effects of sin, we will utilize the healing effect of the leaves of the tree of life as we "grow up as calves of the stall."

God gave Adam and Eve plants to eat of in paradise, and the wonderful "green herb" even has a central role for our health after we are in heaven! Should we not make the most of this wonderful nutritional gift while we are still here on this earth?

The antediluvian age, that is, the era of history before the flood seems to be a mysterious time as comparatively little is recorded about that period, at least compared to other eras we know of today. Much speculation abounds by those who seek to explain exactly what took place then, but again, that is not the best way to approach gaining an understanding of things. As always, we should use comparative analysis and contextual analysis of Scripture to fully know what happened when seemingly little explanation is given. The prophet Isaiah confirms this: "Whom shall he teach knowledge? and whom shall he make to understand doctrine? ... For precept must be upon precept ... line upon line ... here a little, and there a little" (Isa. 28:9, 10).

So why were we told so little about the times before the flood? Men and women were giants in those days, both physically and mentally. Almost angelic in form, they were much closer in every way to the way God had originally created humanity in His perfection. With their exceedingly great powers of mind and body, we can imagine that the average person then could easily accomplish far more in a short period of time than our greatest geniuses and experts today could accomplish in a lifetime. This, along with the fact that humans today rarely live beyond a century whereas in the antediluvian age the average lifespan was nearly a thousand years, shows us that during that period of earth's history more had been accomplished by humanity than all the books in the entire planet today could contain! No doubt Satan himself was very pleased indeed to be in control of such a powerful race of beings.

The power and understanding of those before the flood was not only that of body and intellect, but they had an understanding of spiritual matters far beyond that of any humans since. The Garden of Eden was still upon the earth in those days, and man offered daily sacrifices at its eastern gate. The gate was guarded by cherubim and a "flaming sword which turned every way," keeping sinful humanity from entering and eating from the tree of life (Gen. 3:24). Neither was there any need for holy writings as there is today, as righteous men, with their great mental powers, accurately stored centuries of detailed knowledge in their memories to be passed on from generation to generation. Everyone knew who the one true God was. Even guilty Cain, after brutally murdering his brother, Abel, spoke with God when He questioned him about his crime and the whereabouts of Abel.

The entire earth was far more beautiful and habitable than it is today as it had not yet suffered the devastating affects of the flood. Both the weather and the geography were virtually a picture of paradise. There was no rain in that time; the ground was, instead, watered by a mist that came up from the earth in the evenings (Gen. 2:6). Great beasts also dwelt on the earth then that if they had survived the flood, human beings, in their weakened and degenerated state, would not have been able to control. The total destruction of these powerful creatures during the great deluge upon the earth was simply another act of God's love and mercy for us. Our great God is constantly looking out for us.

Let there be no doubt that in spite of all these showings of mercy by God upon the human race, humanity is still under a worldwide death sentence. We are not born saved. We are all born under sin, and the only way out is to personally choose to be saved in Christ. Truly, "the wages of sin is death" (Rom. 6:23), and "all have sinned, and come short of the glory of God" (Rom. 3:23). We do not naturally deserve life. We should always remember that every breath, every heartbeat, and every thought is a gift from God—a gift not to be taken lightly.

Human history is a long story of God trying to prepare us to be reincorporated back into His kingdom. We are being tested and tried. We should not complain of our problems, for we are very blessed just to be alive. As the wise man, Solomon, said, "For to him that is joined to all the living there is hope: for a living dog is better than a dead lion" (Eccl. 9:4).

Even though before the flood people lived in a near-ideal environment for working, raising children, and worshipping God, a spirit began to creep into the human race, one that could be traced back to the rebelliousness and hatefulness of Cain. Humanity quickly began to populate the earth, and as rebelliousness increased, people began to separate into various tribes and sects. They began to worship nature in place of God, and thus the beginnings of sun-worship entered the world. People also began to worship idols made of stone, wood, and precious metals, not wanting to face the only true God, but blindly worshipping and praying to mute images, which in the end would never hold them accountable.

In Genesis 6 we read: "And it came to pass, when men began to multiply on the face of the earth, and daughters were born unto them, That the sons of God saw the daughters of men that they were fair; and they took them wives of all which they chose. And the Lord said, My spirit shall not always strive with man, for that he also is flesh: yet his days shall be an hundred and twenty years" (Gen. 6:1–3).

Thus God points out to the rapidly multiplying human race, that they would have a probation period of 120 years to turn back from their wickedness. "There were giants in the earth in those days; and also after that, when the sons of God came in unto the daughters of men, and they bare children to them, the same became mighty men which were of old, men of renown. And God saw that the wickedness of man was great in the earth, and that every imagination of the thoughts of his heart was only evil continually. And it repented the Lord that he had made man on the earth, and it grieved him at his heart. And the Lord said, I will destroy man whom I have created from the face of the earth; both man, and beast, and the creeping thing, and the fowls of the air; for it repenteth me that I have made them " (verses 4–7).

Yet in spite of it all, hope was not completely lost, for as we are told, "Noah found grace in the eyes of the Lord" (verse 8). God had to institute a plan for maintaining the purity of the human race if there was to be a coming Redeemer. Noah and his family were literally the last hope for the human race to prolong humanity's existence before they turned themselves completely over to Satan and destroyed themselves.

The story continues in Genesis 6: "The earth also was corrupt before God, and the earth was filled with violence. And God looked upon the earth, and, behold, it was corrupt; for all flesh had corrupted his way upon the earth. And God said unto Noah, The end of all flesh is come before me; for the earth is filled with violence through them; and, behold, I will destroy them with the earth" (verses 11–13).

Then God outlined a plan to Noah: "Make thee an ark ..." (verse 14). So Noah's 120-year mission was to build this gigantic ark so that mankind and all basic life forms on earth could survive the flood and continue on. But the unavoidable concern was that wickedness would spring up again. This was a valid question for which God had a good answer. You see, even though God had intentionally given human beings a nutrient-rich diet in order to increase their lifespan and strength, which was necessary at the time, He now had to decrease their time on earth because before the flood people had become too powerful for their own good.

Do you remember the saying, "Power corrupts, and absolute power corrupts absolutely"? Well this is exactly what had happened to the antediluvian people, and they had to be chastised for their abuse of the gifts God had given them, or else, everything bad that happened before the flood would quickly happen again. Remember, humanity's first "curse" given to them by God was actually a "bailout plan" designed for their own good? Well, now, God had a second type of plan, but it was very opposite in nature.

After the traumatizing experience of the flood had passed and the door of the ark opened, Noah must have been shocked and horrified at what the earth looked like. Everything looked like a vast battlefield with no boundaries—a gigantic wasteland spread out before him. Entire forests had been ripped up by their roots, and even mountains had been moved out of their places. Despair literally filled his heart. Though he knew it to be his home planet, it no longer bore any resemblance to the world he had lived upon for centuries.

Yet, in spite of it all, Noah knew that God had led him this far and that He would not let him down. At this point God blessed Noah and his sons and said unto them, "Be fruitful, and multiply, and replenish the earth" (Gen. 9:1). Therefore, God commanded them to repopulate the world in the very way that their predecessors, Adam and Eve, were told to do centuries before.

In the next two verses, we shall see God's second bailout plan: "And the fear of you and the dread of you shall be upon every beast of the earth, and upon every fowl of the air, upon all that moveth upon the earth, and upon all the fishes of the sea; into your hand are they delivered. Every moving thing that liveth shall be meat for you; even as the green herb have I given you all things" (verses 2, 3).

So now, in addition to the ideal diet of fruits, seeds, and herbs, humanity was given permission to eat the flesh of the beasts of the earth as well. Eating flesh did not lawfully begin when Adam and Eve were cast out of Eden, but only after the Great Flood.

Even though all the vegetation on the earth had been destroyed by the deluge, This was the primary reason why He gave Noah and his family flesh to eat. God could have given them "bread from heaven" as He did with the Israelites in the wilderness, if He pleased, but that was not part of His plan. Why? There was indeed a method to this seeming madness.

And just as the Lord had given the human race green herbs and hard labor as a prescription for extending their life before, He now had to shorten the lives of humanity or else the same evils that led to their downfall before would overtake them a second time. It was this purpose that led to the addition of animal flesh to their diet. This must have been very difficult for Noah, because to him the very thought of eating a piece of flesh, whether that of a cow, a chicken, or a fish, would have been utterly repugnant to him. But being he was a true man of God, he did what he was told to do.

All this being considered, human beings were not given an open license to eat anything and everything that dwelt upon the earth. Unclean beasts were forbidden as food, which is why God told Noah to take "every clean beast ... by sevens, the male and his female: and of beasts that are not clean by two, the male and his female" (Gen. 7:2).

Leviticus 11 and Deuteronomy 14 give more details on the difference between clean and unclean animals. These laws are health-based, as many of the creatures that are forbidden to eat, such as the swine and shellfish, feed upon every detestable thing, and their bodies are filled with disease, toxic substances, and parasites. These laws began with Noah, not with Abraham or Moses. Although Jews follow these teachings, they are universal health principles that apply to all people. Consuming fat and blood was also prohibited. As God said to Noah after He gave him flesh to eat: "But flesh with the life thereof, which is the blood thereof, shall ye not eat" (Gen. 9:4). And again, to the Israelites, He said, "It shall be a perpetual statute for your generations throughout all your dwellings, that ye eat neither fat nor blood" (Lev. 3:17).

Nearly everyone today knows that eating animal fat is not good for you in any amount, but the blood is also very unhealthful as it begins to putrefy in the animal's flesh very quickly after it is slaughtered. The results of putrefaction are highly toxic and dangerous to one's health. However, for the true flesh-eating addict, the fat and blood would be difficult to give up, as that is what gives the flesh its flavor and texture. Kosher meat, which has all the fat and blood removed, is known to be tough and tasteless, thereby needing a lot of seasoning and tenderizing to make it palatable. But in spite of all these careful restrictions on eating flesh to minimize its unhealthful effects, it still served its purpose very well—it shortened people's lifespan and weakened their vital force.

Every generation before the flood, from Adam to Noah, lived just short of a thousand years. But after meat entered the diet, every generation after Noah began to steadily decline in the total number of years lived. Even though Noah, the ninth generation from Adam, outlived Adam by twenty years, Abraham, a righteous man called by God to father the nation of Israel, was ten generations after Noah and only lived to be 175, which if you do the math is 775 years less than Noah.

But God had a new bailout plan to get His people back on track.

When God first called Abraham, who was then called Abram, to be the father of His new nation, He told him, "Get thee out of thy country, and from thy kindred, and from thy father's house, unto a land that I will shew thee: And I will make of thee a great nation, and I will bless thee, and make thy name great; and thou shalt be a blessing: And I will bless them that bless thee, and curse him that curseth thee: and in thee shall all families of the earth be blessed" (Gen. 12:1–3).

Note that the blessing promised by God to Abraham was to be universal for all peoples of the world to benefit from—"and in thee shall all families of the earth be blessed." Even the wicked are blessed by the presence of the righteous, whether they acknowledge and appreciate it or not. When Jesus gave His famous Sermon on the Mount, He was speaking almost entirely to Jews, the sons and daughters of Israel. To them He said, "Ye are the light of the world. A city that is set on an hill cannot be hid. Neither do men light a candle, and put it under a bushel, but on a candlestick; and it giveth light unto all that are in the house. Let your light so shine before men, that they may see your good works, and glorify your Father which is in heaven" (Matt. 5:14–16).

This is what God originally commissioned the Jewish people to do. To be a beacon of righteousness upon the earth that all people from all nations would be drawn to and receive the blessings thereby. The nation of Israel began with Abraham and grew until it was made up of twelve tribes: "Abraham begat Isaac; and Isaac begat Jacob [later called Israel]; and Jacob begat Judas and his brethren" (Matt. 1:2).

Jacob had twelve sons, but one son, Joseph, was sold into slavery in Egypt (Gen. 39). Through a series of divine events that are documented in Genesis chapters 40 through 50, Joseph becomes a high-ranking official in Pharaoh's court and eventually is reunited with his family. Joseph's entire family settles in the land of Goshen, and they and their descendants prospered. "And Joseph died, and all his brethren, and all that generation. And the children of Israel were fruitful, and increased abundantly, and multiplied, and waxed exceeding mighty; and the land was filled with them" (Exod. 1:6, 7).

But this is when troubles began. "Now there arose up a new king over Egypt, which knew not Joseph. And he said unto his people, Behold, the people of the children of Israel are more and mightier than we: Come on, let us deal wisely with them; lest they multiply, and it come to pass, that, when there falleth out any war, they join also unto our enemies, and fight against us, and so get them up out of the land. Therefore they did set over them taskmasters to afflict them with their burdens. And they built for Pharaoh treasure cities, Pithom and Raamses. But the more they afflicted them, the more they multiplied and grew. And they were grieved because of the children of Israel.... And they made their lives bitter with hard bondage, in mortar, and in brick, and in all manner of service in the field: all their service, wherein they made them serve, was with rigour" (Exod. 1:8–14).

God, in order to release His children from Egyptian bondage and lead them into the Promised Land (both literally and spiritually), had to come up with a third "bailout plan." So He sent them a man to lead them. Moses followed God's commands and went before Pharaoh and said, "Let my people go" (Exod. 5:1). Even though these words are central to the story, getting the children of Israel out of Egypt really wasn't the hard part. Getting them into the Promised Land was the really hard part!

God's promise to Israel that they would inherit a land flowing with milk and honey rested entirely upon whether or not the nation would obey His commandments and keep His laws. While the exodus from Egypt took place relatively quickly, the long, bitter forty-year journey in the wilderness was full of tests and trials they did not foresee.

Upon their release from slavery, God began the task of trying to undo years of corruption and learned behaviors that the children of Israel had picked up from the Egyptians. So He started with the very basics. He gave them His law written upon tablets of stone—the very foundation upon which the government of God itself is based. Every sin known to humanity is a violation of one or more of these ten laws. As our Master, Jesus, taught, even the very thoughts of the heart are included (Matt. 5:21–28).

Scripture teaches that "sin is the transgression of the law" (1 John 3:4), but by the power of love in our hearts, we fulfill the law (Rom. 13:10). As Jesus said, "If ye love me, keep my commandments" (John 14:15). To be saved in Christ, we need the law. Why? Because "by the law is the knowledge of sin" (Rom. 3:20), and without the knowledge of sin, how can we admit to God we are sinners who are under a death sentence and need to be saved?

The three basic steps to salvation in Christ are 1) justification, 2) sanctification, 3) glorification. The path of the children of Israel from Egypt through the wilderness and to the Promised Land is an accurate depiction of all three of the essential steps to salvation. Israel passing through the Red Sea soon after their release from captivity symbolizes justification through Christ. The blood on the doorposts represented the blood of Christ, and the Passover lamb represented Him as "the Lamb of God, which taketh away the sins of the world" (John 1:29). This was purely an act of God's grace. We cannot justify ourselves before God. This can only be done through the blood of Christ and His sacrifice for us.

Just as the process of sanctification, being sanctified or "set apart" before God, begins immediately after we are justified in Christ, so the journey of the Israelites in the wilderness began after they crossed the Red Sea. They could not be taken immediately into the Promised Land because of their spiritual condition. It was because of their own wickedness that they had to wander for forty years in that desolate land before receiving God's promise.

Their situation was identical to that of the church in Laodicea, the last of the seven, which represents God's people in the last days of earth's history. To them He wrote, "Because thou sayest, I am rich, and increased with goods, and have need of nothing; and knowest not that thou art wretched, and miserable, and poor, and blind, and naked" (Rev. 3:17). Just as with Laodicea, Israel was not truly aware of their real spiritual condition. They had lived in spiritual blindness for so long, just going along with the flow of the world around them, that they had come to think they were just fine the way they were! They did not know that they had to be "tried in the fire" (Rev. 3:18) and tested by the Holy Spirit in order to receive glorification, which is eternal life with God in heaven! How few people in the world today, even among Christians who claim to keep "the commandments of God, and have the testimony of Jesus Christ" (Rev. 12:17), really understand the true ways of the King of the universe!

Let us continue on. The majority of people everywhere just assume that the law of God, the Ten Commandments, is just a basic set of moral principles that pretty much applies to every civilized land and nation around the world. Yet while very few really know the commandments by heart, they think they know and understand what they represent, and they believe that that's good enough. Most people come to this conclusion based upon the "shortened" versions they may have seen in a movie or on large tablets of stone standing in prominent public places or on the walls of their church. But this is part of Satan's deception. He does not want people to know what God's complete standard of sin is, because our adversary, the devil, does not want anyone entering His kingdom, and the knowledge of sin is the first step to being saved.

As the apostle James tells us: "For whosoever shall keep the whole law, and yet offend in one point, he is guilty of all. For he that said, Do not commit adultery, said also, Do not kill. Now if thou commit no adultery, yet if thou kill, thou art become a transgressor of the law. So speak ye, and so do, as they that shall be judged by the law of liberty" (James 2:10–12).

Again, let us hear the words of Christ on this matter: "Think not that I am come to destroy the law, or the prophets: I am not come to destroy, but to fulfil. For verily I say unto you, Till heaven and earth pass, one jot or one tittle shall in no wise pass from the law, till all be fulfilled. Whosoever therefore shall break one of these least commandments, and shall teach men so, he shall be called the least in the kingdom of heaven: but whosoever shall do and teach them, the same shall be called great in the kingdom of heaven" (Matt. 5:17–19).

All this considered, did you know that there is an almost universally "forgotten commandment"? It is actually one of the ten that almost nobody knows about, and people who have a passing familiarity with it don't even know what it stands for. Sound crazy? It is, but it gets even crazier! The very commandment that has been most forgotten and put aside as unimportant is actually the most important of them all because it identifies just who and what God is! We can only worship God if we know who He is. As Jesus taught, the answer is found in the beginning.

In the Bible the Ten Commandments are found in Exodus 20:3-17. Only one of the ten perfectly identifies who and what God is. It is the fourth commandment, which is also known as the seal of God. So just what is a seal? In ancient times, a seal was found on a ring usually worn by a ruler, such as a king. A seal identified the ruler in three ways, for inscribed on it was 1) his name, 2) his title, and 3) his territory.

Now let's examine the fourth commandment in the Deca-logue, which shows us all of the aspects of a seal: "Remember the sabbath day, to keep it holy. Six days shalt thou labour, and do all thy work: But the seventh day is the sabbath of the Lord thy God: in it thou shalt not do any work, thou, nor thy son, nor thy daughter, thy manservant, nor thy maidservant, nor thy cattle, nor thy stranger that is within thy gates: For in six days the Lord made heaven and earth, the sea, and all that in them is, and rested the seventh day: wherefore the Lord blessed the sabbath day, and hal-lowed it" (Exod. 20:8–11).

So just what do we see here in the fourth commandment that shows God's seal? It is as follows: 1) His name is "thy God," 2) His title is "the Lord," and 3) His territory is "heaven and earth, the sea, and all that in them is." As with other truths, God takes us back to the beginning of creation to show us just who and what He is. The reminder of the Sabbath is founded in Creation before the fall. It tells us in Genesis: "Thus the heavens and the earth were finished, and all the host of them. And on the seventh day God ended his work which he had made; and he rested on the seventh day from all his work which he had made. And God blessed the seventh day, and sanctified it: because that in it he had rested from all his work which God created and made" (Gen. 2:1–3).

The fact is that we cannot really worship God unless we do so in "spirit and in truth" (John 4:24). And the truth only comes from an understanding of the Word of God. No amount of meditation or staring at the stars will give you that truth! This is not just about basic morality, for even the basest of sinners can show some level of that, which Jesus speaks of: "For if ye love them which love you, what reward have ye? do not even the publicans the same? And if ye salute your brethren only, what do ye more than others? do not even the publicans so? Be ye therefore perfect, even as your Father which is in heaven is perfect" (Matt. 5:46–48).

When God seeks out His people who are lost, the first thing He shows them is who He is—their Creator. Let us look at the apostle Paul's tactics when preaching to the paganistic Greeks in the city of Athens. "Ye men of Athens, I perceive that in all things ye are too superstitious. For as I passed by, and beheld your devotions, I found an altar with this inscription, TO THE UNKNOWN GOD. Whom therefore ye ignorantly worship, him declare I unto you" (Acts 17:22, 23).

Then Paul declared the "unknown" God, who is the true God, to the Athenians. "God that made the world and all things therein, seeing that he is Lord of heaven and earth ... seeing he giveth to all life, and breath, and all things; And hath made of one blood all nations of men for to dwell on all the face of the earth, and hath determined the times before appointed, and the bounds of their habitation; That they should seek the Lord, if haply they might feel after him, and find him, though he be not far from every one of us: For in him we live, and move, and have our being; as certain also of your own poets have said, For we are also his offspring" (verses 24–29).

Why did Paul start with God's creatorship? Because if He were not our Creator, He could not be our Savior! Christ had to not only suffer the death penalty for our sins in order to save us, but He had to survive the bottomless pit of the grave in order for us to survive eternal death. Christ, therefore, had to be fully human to be put to death, but He also had to be fully divine in order to be resurrected from the grave. No created being, not even a sinless angel from heaven, could have done this. The justice of God demands eternal death as the consequences for all sin; Christ is both our Creator and the sacrifice for our sins. Hallelujah!

Now we shall delve into how God's true people are to honor our Creator and Savior.

At the beginning, our Lord established three identifying marks for His holy people, all of which were given in the Garden of Eden before Adam and Eve disobeyed God. They are as follows: 1) the seal of God, 2) the marriage seal, and 3) the original diet.

The seal of God, His holy Sabbath day, was established as an eternal reminder of God's act of creating the world in six days and resting on the seventh day. The prophet Isaiah tells us how we will regard the Sabbath in heaven and the new earth. "For as the new heavens and the new earth, which I will make, shall remain before me, saith the Lord, so shall your seed and your name remain. And it shall come to pass, that from one new moon to another, and from one sabbath to another, shall all flesh come to worship before me, saith the Lord" (Isa. 66:22, 23). (Note: We can most likely assume that the festival of the new moon was not only a Jewish ceremonial holiday, as those listed in Leviticus 23, but was also established in Eden, as was the Sabbath, and was made for all humanity to observe, but only while they had access to the tree of life. It is very likely that the new moon was a monthly festival that coincides with the bearing of the "twelve manner of fruits" of the tree of life, which yields "her fruit every month" as mentioned in Revelation 22:2.)

Let us remember that God was not tired when He rested on the seventh day after creating the world. He made it for our blessing, As Jesus said, "The sabbath was made for man, and not man for the sabbath" (Mark 2:27). We are to receive nothing but blessings by observing God's holy memorial for His creative act, and so shall it be throughout eternity. The seven-day week has remained a constant ever since our Lord instituted it at Creation, as documented in Genesis chapters 1 and 2. To know how to keep the Lord's Sabbath day properly, all we need to do is to claim the promise in the Scripture that states "seek, and ye shall find" (Matt. 7:7).

Christ's sheep always hear His voice. We have seen both in this and the previous chapters that in order for God to fully reestablish His people as a "light of the world" (Matt. 5:14), He must show them, first and foremost, just who and what He is to them. Thus, the Sabbath and the Ten Commandments were given as a seal of His creatorship to Christ's followers.

But the Lord also knew too well that they would not be faithful and obedient to Him unless He literally nipped the very source of all unlawful desires at the bud. This wicked root that all other branches of human desire spring forth from is the appetite.

Appetite is the original sin of mankind, and not just symbolically or historically. It is literally at the heart of all other human passions and desires, which constantly draws people away from God. As small and insignificant as this human passion may seem to us, it is truly the tiny spark that begins an entire forest fire.

Returning the Israelites to the original diet God had given humanity in the beginning was an essential part of preparing them to be His holy nation. The flesh diet had fully played its role in shortening the lives of everyone. Now, it was time to restore His people to the plan He had given them at Creation, that they may be completely brought back to an ideal state of body, mind, and spiritual state of being, and that through them, all may know who the mighty God of heaven and earth truly is. To accomplish this, God designed a test for Israel, one that would teach both the lessons of His holy Sabbath and that of controlling human appetite. In order to do this, He denied them the delicacies of Egypt that they had become so accustomed to, and in its place, He gave them manna, which is referred to as "bread from heaven" (Exod. 16:4).

Exodus 16 chronicles the story of the Israelites, and the Sabbath test in which they were instructed to collect double the amount needed on Friday to last through Sabbath. But on no other day of the week could they collect double; for if they kept it overnight, it would spoil. Then in Numbers 11 we find the story of the quail. Because they begged for meat, God gave them what they wanted, and they suffered the consequences of their untamed appetite.

Now let's look at the seriousness of this matter, according to the consult of Solomon: "And put a knife to thy throat, if thou be a man given to appetite" (Prov. 23:2). Now turn to Philippians 3:18, 19 and see what Paul wrote to the church of Philippi: "For many walk, of whom I have told you often, and now tell you even weeping, that they are the enemies of the cross of Christ: Whose end is destruction, whose God is their belly, and whose glory is in their shame, who mind earthly things."

If we are not to be counted as "enemies of the cross of Christ," then we must avoid making our belly into a false idol before God, for it would be better to "put a knife to thy throat" than to do otherwise. There are three steps that lead us into utter corruption: 1) appetite, 2) lust, and 3) anger, and appetite is the most subtle of all temptations.

Consider the very first temptation. "Now the serpent was more subtil than any beast of the field which the Lord God had made. And he said unto the woman, Yea, hath God said, Ye shall not eat of every tree of the garden? And the woman said unto the serpent, We may eat of the fruit of the trees of the garden: But of the fruit of the tree which is in the midst of the garden, God hath said, Ye shall not eat of it, neither shall ye touch it, lest ye die. And the serpent said unto the woman, Ye shall not surely die" (Gen. 3:1–3). This was the very first lie ever declared to humanity by the great deceiver, Satan, that people could live forever and ever, throughout all eternity, even if they chose to disobey God.

And so the subtle serpent continues on in his first great deception of humanity. "For God doth know that in the day ye eat thereof, then your eyes shall be opened, and ye shall be as gods, knowing good and evil" (verse 5). So in addition to the promise of immortality apart from God, he offers to her another aspect of achieving a godlike nature—that of a knowledge which God has been holding back from them. Thus, the breeding of distrust and lack of faith in God was central to his great lie. In other words, "Don't believe what God tells you. I've got something far better!"

And just what was the key to this demonic equation? Continue reading: "And when the woman saw that the tree was good for food, and that it was pleasant to the eyes, and a tree to be desired to make one wise, she took of the fruit thereof, and did eat, and gave also unto her husband with her; and he did eat" (verse 6).

Thus we see that the "entering wedge" to the human heart in this first sin was appetite. This is because the appetite is the great enticer that opens up the door for all other sins to enter in. Once the unlawful appetite is indulged, then comes lust, and not just that of a sexual nature, although sexually-based lust is included. Lust is simply a desire for things that God has forbidden. As the apostle said. "For I had not known lust, except the law had said, Thou shalt not covet" (Rom. 7:7). John also wrote, saying, "For all that is in the world, the lust of the flesh, and the lust of the eyes, and the pride of life, is not of the Father, but is of the world" (1 John 2:16).

Here we can clearly see that the human appetite, when we allow it to entice us to indulgence, automatically becomes uncontrolled, which then leads to uncontrolled lusts of various kinds. When these base and worldly passions and desires are not allowed to vent themselves, outright rage is the inevitable result. Satan himself is the epitome, the personification, of this rage in his very nature. "Be sober, be vigilant; because your adversary the devil, as a roaring lion, walketh about, seeking whom he may devour" (1 Peter 5:8).

Thus we see that appetite entices us, which leads to lust that overwhelms us, which then leads to anger that consumes us. The more these perverted instincts are given sway in our daily lives, the more we thereby distance ourselves from our Creator. This is why God wanted to show the children of Israel in the wilderness a better way. God wanted to show His holy people the wonderful graces given at Creation that would seal them as His very own. Thus He gave them manna, a perfect food in every way. The manna appeared in the camp each night so that in the morning the Israelites could gather it and use it for both the morning and evening meals. If they attempted to keep any of the manna for the next day, it spoiled and became infested with worms. But as mentioned, on the sixth day of the week (the preparation day for the Sabbath), the Lord gave them twice as much since there would be no manna on the ground on the Sabbath. In this manner, the Sabbath lesson was taught to the Israelites.

This, however, was not the big test. Even though the psalmist tells us that they were given "angels' food" to eat in the wilderness (Ps. 78:25), they were very dissatisfied with this perfect diet. "And the whole congregation of the children of Israel murmured against Moses and Aaron in the wilderness: And the children of Israel said unto them, Would to God we had died by the hand of the Lord in the land of Egypt, when we sat by the flesh pots, and when we did eat bread to the full; for ye have brought us forth into this wilderness, to kill this whole assembly with hunger. Then said the Lord unto Moses, Behold, I will rain bread from heaven for you ... that I may prove them, whether they will walk in my law, or no" (Exod. 16:2–4).

The Israelites were not battling with true hunger. Their heavenly diet lacked nothing nutritionally! What they were struggling with was their perverted appetites, particularly, their overwhelming lust for the "flesh pots" of Egypt, which is why God made this a testing point, "whether they will walk in my law, or no."

The book of Numbers gives us more insight into their quest for meat. "And the mixt multitude that was among them fell a lusting: and the children also wept again, and said, Who shall give us flesh to eat?... But now our soul is dried away: there is nothing at all, beside this manna, before our eyes" (Num. 11:4, 6). While the Israelites desired for a variety of foods they had in Egypt, it was the truly harmful addiction, that of animal flesh, that God was trying to break them from, and He knew that if the children of Israel could be disciplined to subsist entirely upon the diet He had given them, all other issues would be much easier to overcome.

However, addictive behavior is never rational, whether it be addiction to food, coffee, cigarettes, alcohol, or drugs. It all springs forth from the same abnormal state of thinking. To the addict, that which is healthy is never "good enough" for them. There is always that ravenous craving, that irrational voice inside their head saying, "I must have it!" Is fresh air good enough for the habitual cigarette smoker? Is a glass of water enough to please a hardened alcoholic? Well, neither was God's original diet enough for those whose hearts and minds still resided in Egypt. But God knew how difficult the transition was for His people; thus He allowed for a temporary compromise, not only to show that He was reasonable but to give them a little time to "wean" them from their dietary addictions.

Still, He was not happy with their stubborn rebelliousness, of which He let them know, as we see in the following verses: "Sanctify yourselves against to morrow, and ye shall eat flesh: for ye have wept in the ears of the Lord, saying, Who shall give us flesh to eat? for it was well with us in Egypt: therefore the Lord will give you flesh, and ye shall eat. Ye shall not eat one day, nor two days, nor five days, neither ten days, nor twenty days; But even a whole month, until it come out at your nostrils, and it be loathsome unto you" (Num. 11:18–20).

So the Lord arranged to give the Israelites quails to eat in the evening while He still gave them manna in the mornings. But what was the final result of this compromise? It was basically the same as in all other instances where God allows His people to go against what He knows to be best for them. "And while the flesh was yet between their teeth, ere it was being chewed, the wrath of the Lord was kindled against the people, and the Lord smote the people with a very great plague. And he called the name of that place Kibrothhattaavah: because there they buried the people that lusted" (verses 33, 34).

But while it goes without saying that any deviation from the laws of nature and health are going to inevitably lead to sickness, it is obvious here that the Israelites were punished for more than just eating what God allowed them to temporarily have. It is most likely that in their maddened state of thinking, that as very soon after they saw the quails, they violated God's health principles and neglected to remove the fat and blood from the flesh of the quails. The plague that fell upon those "that lusted" was certainly no act of cruelty on God's part. As we shall see throughout this book, God has indeed allowed His people compromises at times to temporarily accommodate them, but the end result of these compromises of principles always result in evil.

Paul the apostle writes to us that the experiences of Israel in the wilderness are examples that we should learn from, and not repeat, particularly for those of us "upon whom the ends of the world are come" (1 Cor. 10:11). He wrote, "Moreover, brethren, I would not that ye should be ignorant, how that our fathers were under the cloud, and all passed through the sea; And were all baptized unto Moses in the cloud and in the sea; And did all eat the same spiritual meat; And did all drink the same spiritual drink: for they drank of that spiritual Rock that followed them: and that Rock was Christ. But with many of them God was not well pleased: for they were overthrown in the wilderness. Now these things were our examples, to the intent we should not lust after evil things, as they also lusted.... Neither murmur ye, as some of them also murmured, and were destroyed of the destroyer. Now all these things happened unto them for examples: and they are written for out admonition, upon whom the ends of the world are come. Wherefore let him that thinketh he standeth take heed lest he fall" (1 Cor. 10:1–12).

Needless to say, the experiences of the Israelites are by no means just "dead history" with no application beyond when it happened. We see that their experiences are very much living examples for us in the here and now. Thus far we have seen how God, in order to prepare His people to enter the Promised Land, sought to restore in them the "three links"—the Sabbath, the marriage bond, and the original diet—in the chain of His eternal creation standard.

We have briefly discussed the Sabbath and diet, but now let's look at marriage. Regarding marriage, it was the case in Israelite culture, as in the surrounding nations, to practice polygamy. Although not part of God's ideal plan, it was widely accepted as the norm. It was so thoroughly ingrained in the practices and thinking of the people that the average male (not to mention one of greatly increased wealth and political power) would have found the very idea of being bound to a single female for his entire life abhorrent.

Even in the time of Christ, 1,500 years after Moses, this way of living was still widely accepted. Read the following exchange between Christ and the Pharisees regarding marriage. "The Pharisees also came unto him, tempting him, and saying unto him, Is it lawful for a man to put away his wife for every cause? And he answered and said unto them, Have ye not read, that he which made them at the beginning made them male and female, And said, For this cause shall a man leave father and mother, and shall cleave to his wife: and they twain shall be one flesh? Wherefore they are no more twain, but one flesh. What therefore God hath joined together, let not man put asunder" (Matt. 19:3–6).

Christ's argument makes sense, right? No Christian questions our Master's logic regarding the sanctity of the marriage bond. But that was not the end of the discussion, for the Pharisees had an "ace in their hand" that they threw at Christ. "Why did Moses then command to give a writing of divorcement, and to put her away?" (verse 7). No Jewish person in Christ's day questioned the absolute spiritual authority of the laws of Moses, and they quoted straight from the book of Deuteronomy, chapter 24 to be exact. What possible answer could Jesus give them on this? They thought they had Him on this one.

But Jesus replied, "Moses because of the hardness of your hearts suffered you to put away your wives"—and now Jesus plays His ace—"but from the beginning it was not so" (verse 8). Even Jesus' own disciples had a hard time swallowing this one, as they said to Him, "If the case of the man be so with his wife, it is not good to marry" (verse 10).

Jesus did not contradict the laws of Moses. Instead, He proclaimed, "Think not that I am come to destroy the law, or the prophets: I am not come to destroy, but to fulfil. For verily I say unto you, Till heaven and earth pass, one jot or one tittle shall in no wise pass from the law, till all be fulfilled" (Matt. 5:17, 18). What Jesus showed everyone here is that all the temporary and imperfect "handwriting of ordinances that was against us, which was contrary to us" (Col. 2:14), "which stood only in ... carnal ordinances, imposed on them until the time of reformation" (Heb. 9:10) was to be removed and nailed to the cross of Christ forever.

All the while, the perfect eternal standards established at Creation and reaffirmed in the Ten Commandments was to be shown in its true glory through Him. The laws of Moses are filled with compromises that were allowed only because of the "hardness of your hearts," all of which had to be swept away before the plan of salvation could be made complete.

The "time of reformation" spoken of in Hebrews began when Christ started His ministry on this earth. Although God allowed His true standard of marriage to be "put on hold" in the days of Israel under the Mosaic law, it had to be put back into its true light before the Lamb of God, who took away the sins of the world, was to be slain on the cross. Why? Because there is more to marriage than what meets the eye. This is why Christ, when He began His ministry on earth with His well-known Sermon on the Mount, made sure there were no misunderstandings regarding marriage (see Matt. 5:31, 32).

The joining of a man and a woman in matrimony has a much deeper meaning than what we see on the surface. It literally symbolizes the relationship between Christ and His holy church. It is for this reason that Satan hates the sanctity of the marriage bond more than anything else imaginable. He tries to destroy it with all his might, as it is the very representation on earth of the relationship between Christ and His people. The more our enemy can deface this sacred tie, the more he can prevent God's true glory from being shown on this earth. Paul reaffirms this truth to the Ephesians: "For we are members of his body, of his flesh, and of his bones. For this cause shall a man leave his father and mother, and shall be joined unto his wife, and they two shall be one flesh. This is a great mystery: but I speak concerning Christ and the church" (Eph. 5:30–32). Along with this "great mystery," Paul tells us the secret to a perfect marriage: "Nevertheless let every one of you in particular so love his wife even as himself; and the wife see that she reverence her husband" (verse 33).

It should be noted here that husbands should remember that whenever there is a disagreement they should not rule their household with an iron hand, but rather should be as Christ is to us, His church, and give "honour unto the wife, as unto the weaker vessel, and as being heirs together of the grace of life; that your prayers be not hindered" (1 Peter 3:7). In Scripture, Christ is referred to as the Bridegroom, and we, the church, are His bride. This is why in Bible prophecy a pure, holy woman represents the church of Christ, whereas an adulterous whore represents a false church that serves Satan (Rev. 12 and 17).

We, as God's people, are now being called to represent Him on earth as a church, as married couples and families, and as individuals. Before all of the saints of God can be completely renewed in mankind's original glory, God must restore all of His holy standards among His representatives on earth. He must show the universe that it can and will be done in spite of humanity's previous wickedness. Of this we may claim the promise "I can do all things through Christ which strengtheneth me" (Phil. 4:13) and know that God will not give us more than we are able to bear (John 16:12).

Only by following the Creation standard can we successfully represent Christ and be glorified on this earth.

When the nation of Israel reached its pinnacle of power and glory under King David and King Solomon, they were many centuries removed from the days of Moses. Under the rule of these righteous men of God, Israel prospered as had been promised to them: "And it shall come to pass, if thou shalt hearken diligently unto the voice of the Lord thy God, to observe and to do all his commandments which I command thee this day, that the Lord thy God will set thee on high above all nations of the earth: And all these blessings shall come on thee, and overtake thee, if thou shalt hearken unto the voice of the Lord thy God" (Deut. 28:1, 2).

Israel was established as a great nation upon the earth, and their capital city, Jerusalem, the "City of Peace," was the location of their temple. Also, their king resided in Jerusalem; thus their theocratic government was centered there. However, having a fallen, sinful, and mortal man as their king was never God's ideal for them. This allowance, like so many other compromises, turned into another "Achilles heel" that furthered the fall of His nation. Their desire to follow the pagan ways of the neighboring nations surrounding them, rather than be a "peculiar people" unto God, is what ultimately led to their downfall.

God predicted this in Deuteronomy 17:14: "When thou art come unto the land which the Lord thy God giveth thee, and shalt possess it, and shalt dwell therein, and shalt say, I will set a king over me, like as all the nations that are about me." To assist the Israelite kings in leading wisely, the Lord gave them a set of rules on how they should conduct themselves. If the kings followed these standards and obeyed God, it was promised to them that they would reap the blessings thereof. Unfortunately, the kings who ruled the nation disregarded many of God's guidelines.

But there were those who followed God and looked to Him for direction. Two prominent rulers in Israelite history were David and Solomon. Under his rule, Solomon oversaw the final completion of what would be the most wonderful and majestic temple of the Lord ever seen in Jerusalem. David designed the temple, but since it was not completed and dedicated until after David's passing, it was thereby known as "Solomon's Temple." Its awesome physical beauty and majestic glory was truly a symbol of the blessings Israel as a nation was receiving under God. The temple was completed nearly half a millennia after the first tabernacle was given to Israel through Moses. Had this mighty and wonderful nation continued following God, the blessings would have been poured out upon them, but that was not to be the case.

Four centuries after the dedication of Solomon's glorious temple, it was to be utterly destroyed by the invading forces of the Babylonian nation, which was the offspring of the people of the ancient city of Babel, the name of which means "confusion." Israel was overcome by a nation that had its roots in confusion because Israel itself, by straying from the clear path of the Lord, had entered into spiritual confusion. Remember what we spoke about before on spiritual compromises? Well, it was the compromises that God had reluctantly allowed Israel and the "hardness of their hearts" that ended up paving the way that led from one compromise to another until, little by little, they completely fell away from God and back into paganism as they had in Egypt.

Of the three identifying marks of Creation—the Sabbath, marriage, and the original diet—none were ever wholeheartedly accepted at any point by Israel. Even the great kings of Israel who were familiar with the laws of Moses regarding the way a king should live, in their pride and self-glorying, fell into sin by disregarding the direct commands of God.

The Lord had told all the kings of Israel, "Neither shall he multiply wives to himself, that his heart turn not away: neither shall he greatly multiply to himself silver and gold" (Deut. 17:17). But we know that David and Solomon didn't follow this explicit command. We are told in Scripture that they literally had hundreds of wives and concubines in their personal harems! In the foolishness of their youth and self-importance, their minds were literally consumed by their passions and pride. Needless to say, as David and Solomon aged, they saw the error of their ways and understood the consequences of their foolish mistakes. Thus Psalms and Proverbs reflect this viewpoint and insight.

This may have seemed like a "Golden Age" in the history of the Israelite nation, but the seeds of wickedness were well planted and were already bearing fruit. The only king in a true theocracy is God Himself! That's why fallen human beings cannot bear the burdens of managing God's government nor can they handle the temptations that inevitably befall them with all the power they wield. It inevitably seems that as soon as God's people begin to reap the physical blessings of obedience to Him they become lazy and self-sufficient, thinking they no longer even need God at all. When we have everything we want handed to us on a silver platter, we automatically begin to stop appreciating it! Then the punishment, the inevitable downfall, comes. This was the real reason for "Adam's curse" given in Genesis 3. As Paul wrote to those in Corinth: "Wherefore let him that thinketh he standeth take heed lest he fall" (1 Cor. 10:12).

When Moses was nearing the end of his life, and he saw that the children of Israel were about to enter the Promised Land completely unprepared, he spoke to them about the blessings and curses they would experience based on their response to God. Here are a few of those words of warning as recorded in Deuteronomy 28: "The Lord shall bring thee, and thy king which thou shalt set over thee, unto a nation which neither thou nor thy fathers have known; and there shalt thou serve other gods, wood and stone. And thou shalt become an astonishment, a proverb, and a byword, among all nations whither the Lord shall lead thee" (verses 36, 37). "The Lord shall bring a nation against thee from far, from the end of the earth, as swift as the eagle flieth; a nation whose tongue thou shalt not understand; A nation of fierce countenance, which shall not regard the person of the old, nor shew favour to the young: And he shall eat the fruit of thy cattle, and the fruit of thy land, until thou be destroyed: which also shall not leave thee either corn, wine, or oil, or the increase of thy kine, or flocks of thy sheep, until he have destroyed thee" (verses 49–51).

And just who was this nation to be? While a thorough study of Daniel 2 and 7 would bear much light on this, we can also see much from a cursory examination of the above verses. We know that this is a pagan nation that was previously unknown to Israel and would take the children of Israel as captives to their land, "unto a nation which neither thou nor thy fathers have known; and there shalt thou serve other gods, wood and stone."

We can also deduce that they are from very far away—"a nation against thee from far, from the end of the earth, as swift as the eagle flieth"—and that it would thereby have a foreign language far different from that of the Hebrews—"a nation whose tongue thou shalt not understand"—and it would be a vicious nation, showing no mercy at all—"A nation of fierce countenance, which shall not regard the person ... until he have destroyed thee."

The brutal, pagan, fierce nation of ancient Babylon perfectly fits the description given here by Moses. When Babylon invaded Jerusalem, they not only ransacked the city, but they took hostage anyone they thought might be able to serve them. Then they utterly decimated the majestic temple built by Solomon, using the riches found therein for their own purposes. Since the ark of the covenant, which contains the Ten Commandments, was hidden in an unknown place outside of Jerusalem before the Babylonian invasion, the original tablets of the covenant and the ark remain safe to this day, to be revealed again shortly before our Lord returns, as a testimony for His law and the eternal standards contained therein.

Babylon was the first of a long line of heathen kingdoms to rule human civilization during ancient times. Daniel, a righteous young man who was taken captive during the Babylonian invasion, matured in Babylon and became an advisor for King Nebuchadnezzar, the ruler of Babylon. The king had prophetic dreams regarding the kingdoms of the world that were to come, including Babylon, Medo-Persia, ancient Greece, and then Rome. In the seventh chapter of the book of Daniel, these kingdoms are prophetically described as "four great beasts" coming up out of the sea, "diverse one from another" (Dan. 7:3). In Bible prophecy, a beast represents a kingdom (Dan. 7:17), and the sea represents populated regions of the world (Rev. 17:15).

The first great beast, which was Babylon, was described in Daniel's dream as "a lion, and had eagle's wings," thus showing further how this nation would be the first to decimate Israel with its Satanic ferocity, "because your adversary the devil, as a roaring lion, walketh about, seeking whom he may devour" (1 Peter 5:8). Babylon came upon Israel "from far, from the end of the earth, as swift as the eagle flieth" as Moses had predicted.

Furthermore, it is entirely appropriate that ancient Babylon is used to symbolically describe the ruling false religious power that exercises its world dominance through its political connections and is literally "drunken with the blood of the saints, and with the blood of the martyrs of Jesus" (Rev. 17:6), both during the period of earth's history known as the Dark Ages as well as in the very last days before Christ's second coming.

After Babylon's destructive takeover, Israel as a nation never regained her former glory. But, nonetheless, there was no shortage of spiritual insight and guidance from God through the prophets, men of God who were enlightened by the spirit of prophecy, giving them both words of hope as well as terrible warnings for the consequences of disobedience to the laws of God. There was one prophet in particular that gave the children of Israel everything needed to prepare them for the first advent of the Messiah, but because of the nature of the truths God had revealed, the full meaning of his words were not to be fully understood until the very end of time.

Chapter Six

A BEACON FOR THE FUTURE

During a time of what must have seemed like utter hopelessness for the nation of Israel, God still had a plan to show them it wasn't too late to straighten up their act and get back on the right track. Even though Israel suffered the consequences of being taken over by Babylon for a long time, the experiences and prophetic insights of Daniel, who was taken prisoner during the takeover, has shed much light on world history and the last days. The book of Daniel was written specifically for a certain period of time in human history, and it was "sealed" until this time. Only partial truths, at best, were brought to understanding before the appointed time, and the truths were only revealed to the righteous that prayerfully sought these things out.

The following texts appear in the last chapter of the book of Daniel: "But thou, O Daniel, shut up the words, and seal the book, even to the time of the end: many shall run to and fro, and knowledge shall be increased.... And he said, Go thy way, Daniel: for the words are closed up and sealed till the time of the end" (Dan. 12:4, 9). We know that during this period of the time of the end "many shall run to and fro, and knowledge shall be increased." Have we not seen the incredible increase in transportation, communication, and all types of knowledge in recent years?

Even though the book of Daniel was to be sealed up until our day and time, its sister book in the Bible, Revelation, was not to be sealed as such. It reads, "And he saith unto me, Seal not the sayings of the prophecy of this book: for the time is at hand" (Rev. 22:10). These two great books of symbolic and apocalyptic prophecy, Daniel and Revelation, though they parallel each other in so many ways, were to walk separate paths through human history until fully rejoined by the "knowledge" that "shall be increased" during the last days.

We are currently living in the last days. If you have any doubts, read Matthew 24, and you will find the words Jesus spoke to His disciples when they asked Him, "Tell us, when shall these things be? and what shall be the sign of thy coming, and of the end of the world?" (verse 3). The troublesome times Christ predicted 2,000 years ago are happening right now before our very eyes. We only need to open our eyes and see it for ourselves.

So what unique purpose does the anciently written book of Daniel serve for us in these modern times? Let us start at the beginning with chapter 1. Daniel and his three friends—Hananiah, Mishael, and Azariah—had just been taken captive to Babylon where they were to be trained in the highest Babylonian schools because they were superior young men. The Bible tells us that they were "children in whom was no blemish, but well favoured, and skilful in all wisdom, and cunning in knowledge, and understanding science" (Dan. 1:4). It was determined that they would have "ability in them to stand in the king's palace, and whom they might teach the learning and the tongue of the Chaldeans" (Ibid.).

But there was a test they had to pass in order to prove their absolute faithfulness to God. It was to be the same test given to Adam and Eve in the Garden of Eden; the same test given to Israel when they left Egypt; and the very first point of temptation that Satan tested Jesus upon after His forty-day fast in the wilderness. It was that of humanity's weakest point in our physical nature— that of the appetite. This is always where it begins.

"And the king appointed them a daily provision of the king's meat, and of the wine which he drank: so nourishing them three years, that at the end thereof they might stand before the king" (verse 5). They probably felt an immense amount of pressure to cave in and just eat whatever their captors gave them without question, but Daniel and his friends chose to do otherwise. "But Daniel purposed in his heart that he would not defile himself with the portion of the king's meat, nor with the wine which he drank: therefore he requested of the prince of the eunuchs that he might not defile himself. Now God had brought Daniel into favour and tender love with the prince of the eunuchs" (verses 8, 9).

Chances are, the prince of the eunuchs, who had grown very close to Daniel, would have been willing to accommodate his request, but there was also another issue at hand. "And the prince of the eunuchs said unto Daniel, I fear my lord the king, who hath appointed your meat and your drink: for why should he see your faces worse liking than the children which are of your sort? then shall ye make me endanger my head to the king" (verse 10).

So Daniel, no doubt not wanting to get anyone into serious trouble, proposed a short test. "Prove thy servants, I beseech thee, ten days; and let them give us pulse [fruits and vegetables] to eat, and water to drink. Then let our countenances be looked upon before thee, and the countenances of the children that eat of the portion of the king's meat: and as thou seest, deal with thy servants. So he consented to them in this matter, and proved them ten days. And at the end of the ten days their countenances appeared fairer and fatter in flesh than all the children which did eat the portion of the king's meat. Thus Melzar took away the portion of their meat, and the wine that they should drink; and gave them pulse" (verses 12–16).

The reason why the prince of the eunuchs feared the king's wrath is because it was commonly believed then, as it is now, that a diet of plant-based foods and water alone would not sufficiently nourish them, and they would experience poor health. The "beer and barbeque" mentality we see today was very much like that of ancient Babylon. How wrong they were! If Daniel and his three friends had not previously lived an abstemious lifestyle with a carefully chosen diet, they would not have passed the appetite test. If they had been addicted to the "flesh-pots" as had their ancestors in the wilderness, their reaction would have been the same as those who said, "But now our soul is dried away: there is nothing at all, beside this manna, before our eyes" (Num. 11:6). When foolishly indulged, the subtle, addictive power of the human appetite is very dangerous indeed.

But the story did not end with the ten-day test. It continues: "As for these four children, God gave them knowledge and skill in all learning and wisdom: and Daniel had understanding in all visions and dreams. Now at the end of the days that the king had said he should bring them in, then the prince of the eunuchs brought them in before Nebuchadnezzar. And the king communed with them; and among them all was found none like Daniel, Hananiah, Mishael, and Azariah: therefore stood they before the king. And in all matters of wisdom and understanding, that the king inquired of them, he found them ten times better than all the magicians and astrologers that were in all his realm" (Dan. 1:17–20).

Scripture tells us that they were not only "fairer and fatter in flesh than all the children which did eat the portion of the king's meat" during the ten-day test, but that also they were found to be "ten times better than all the magicians and astrologers that were in his realm." I don't think they "wasted away" on their comparatively "limited" diet!

Daniel 1 is a lesson for those of us in the last days. As God's true followers, we may be physically "trapped" by the circumstances that surround us, but in spite of this, we are to remain faithful to His principles and be a shining light to those around us. The book of Revelation points us to another group that is trapped, but these people don't even know they are trapped in "spiritual Babylon." It is to this group that this message goes to in the last days as spoken of by the apostle John. "Babylon the great is fallen, is fallen, and is become the habitation of devils, and the hold of every foul spirit, and a cage of every unclean and hateful bird.... Come out of her, my people, that ye be not partakers of her sins, and that ye receive not of her plagues" (Rev. 18:2, 4).

To those who are in spiritual Babylon and need to be called out, Jesus said, "And other sheep I have, which are not of this fold: them also I must bring, and they shall hear my voice; and there shall be one fold, and one shepherd" (John 10:16). In His warnings to Israel, He also speaks of these "other sheep" that will come and take their rightful places in God's kingdom. "And I say unto you, That many shall come from the east and west, and shall sit down with Abraham, and Isaac, and Jacob, in the kingdom of heaven. But the children of the kingdom shall be cast out into outer darkness: there shall be weeping and gnashing of teeth" (Matt. 8:11, 12).

In Daniel 4, Nebuchadnezzar relates a dream he had that no one but Daniel, through the power of God, could interpret. The king dreamed of a great and wonderful tree that bore much fruit, and all the creatures of the earth benefited from its presence. But then the tree was cut down, and all the fruit and leaves were scattered, yet the stump and the roots were left in the earth with a band of iron and brass about it. But in the dream the tree was referred to as a man, one who would be given the heart, or mentality, of a beast for seven years. It was a very mysterious dream indeed.

In spite of knowing Daniel's reputation for knowledge, wisdom, and the interpretation of dreams, Nebuchadnezzar first went to his wise men, magicians, astrologers, and soothsayers. But after they all failed in relaying the meaning of the king's dream, he turned again to Daniel. Let us see what Daniel revealed to the king on this matter: "The tree that thou sawest, which grew, and was strong, whose height reached unto the heaven, and the sight thereof to all the earth; Whose leaves were fair, and the fruit thereof much, and in it was meat for all; under which the beasts of the field dwelt, and upon whose branches the fowls of the heaven had their habitation: It is thou, O king, that art grown and become strong: for thy greatness is grown, and reacheth unto heaven, and thy dominion to the end of the earth" (Dan. 4:20–22).

So the tree in the dream is the king and his kingdom, for as we see in Scripture that trees can refer symbolically to these things. Paul, in Romans 11, depicts Israel as an olive tree which any believer in Christ will be grafted onto it while unbelievers are broken off and cast into the fire. John the Baptist, when speaking to the hypocritical Pharisees and Sadducees coming to him for baptism, spoke these words, "O generation of vipers, who hath warned you to flee from the wrath to come? Bring forth therefore fruits meet for repentance: And think not to say within yourselves, We have Abraham to our father: for I say unto you, that God is able of these stones to raise up children unto Abraham. And now also the axe is laid at the root of the trees: therefore every tree which bringeth not forth good fruit is hewn down, and cast into the fire" (Matt. 3:7–10). Malachi also refers to the utter final destruction of the wicked: "And the day that cometh shall burn them up, saith the Lord of hosts, that it shall leave them neither root nor branch" (Mal. 4:1). Satan is the root, and his followers are the branches.

So while God saw Nebuchadnezzar to be a basically "good tree," he had grown excessively proud and arrogant because of his great power and riches (as had many past kings of Israel), and a change had to be made. Thus Daniel continues in his interpretation of the king's dream: "That they shall drive thee from men, and thy dwelling shall be with the beasts of the field, and they shall make thee to eat grass as oxen, and they shall wet thee with the dew of heaven, and seven times [years] shall pass over thee, till thou know that the most High ruleth in the kingdom of men, and giveth it to whomsoever he will. And whereas they commanded to leave the stump of the tree roots; thy kingdom shall be sure unto thee, after that thou shalt have known that the heavens do rule. Wherefore, O king, let my counsel be acceptable unto thee, and break off thy sins by righteousness, and thine iniquities by showing mercy to the poor; if it may be a lengthening of thy tranquility" (Dan. 4:25–27).

No doubt the king was quite unsettled by what Daniel revealed to him in this dream. Daniel had faithfully revealed to him prophetic interpretations in the past. Why should this one be any different? It is most likely that after first hearing the dream interpreted by Daniel that the king probably made an effort to straighten up his life and follow the advice Daniel had given him. But the test of time, as revealed by the words of the king, showed no real change in his attitude. Regarding our words, Jesus spoke: "O generation of vipers, how can ye, being evil, speak good things? for out of the abundance of the heart the mouth speaketh.... But I say unto you, That every idle word that men shall speak, they shall give account thereof in the day of judgment. For by thy words thou shalt be justified, and by thy words thou shalt be condemned" (Matt. 12:34–37).

But what did the king's words show? "At the end of twelve months he walked in the palace of the kingdom of Babylon. The king spake, and said, Is not this great Babylon, that I have built for the house of the kingdom by the might of my power, and for the honour of my majesty?" (Dan. 4:29, 30). With those words, Nebuchadnezzar brought the sentence from his dream down on his head. "While the word was in the king's mouth, there fell a voice from heaven, saying, O king Nebuchadnezzar, to thee it is spoken; The kingdom is departed from thee. And they shall drive thee from men, and thy dwelling shall be with the beasts of the field: they shall make thee to eat grass as oxen, and seven times shall pass over thee, until thou know that the most High ruleth in the kingdom of men, and giveth it to whomsoever he will. The same hour was the thing fulfilled upon Nebuchadnezzar: and he was driven from men, and did eat grass as oxen, and his body was wet with the dew of heaven, till his hair was grown like eagle's feathers, and his nails like bird's claws" (Dan. 4:31–33).

So, what actual purpose did this strange punishment of King Nebuchadnezzar actually serve? It was no random act on God's part. Scripture shows us that when human beings begin to rebel against God, they become self-serving and starts to create things of their own works in which to glorify themselves. Nebuchadnezzar had become a very proud man, and if God were to purify him from this, it would be no small act. To reach down into the depths of King Nebuchadnezzar's heart and show him how his own unjustified sense of self-worth was actually a festering cancer growing within him, God had to "chastise" the king for seven years in a sentence that actually had its roots in Adam's curse.

When we fall to our lowest depths, but still have a chance to be saved, God brings us back to our beginnings—that is, nature. King Nebuchadnezzar, like the rest of Babylonian culture, thought that overindulgence was the norm and that living a life in harmony with nature was overly restrictive and actually unnatural in itself. When in reality, it is indulgence that clouds the mind and blunts the normal sensibilities, and our natural instincts thereby become perverted to the point that they do not even resemble the instincts that God gave us at Creation. We cannot really know who and what we are and what God really meant for us to be until we are living a life in harmony with the laws of nature. Because God knew that the king had become warped by his own pride and passions, the way He could heal him was to literally give him the mind of a beast for seven years, whereas he lived in a field and ate grass as the oxen.

This is a repeat of what took place in Genesis when God took the food that was originally intended for the beasts, the green herb, and after the fall made it a permanent addition to humanity's diet (Gen. 1:30; 3:18). Yes, this may sound like an extreme measure on God's part, but you can rest assured that it was in no wise unnecessary.

So, at the end of the trial of seven years, what was the king's reaction? "And at the end of the days I Nebuchadnezzar lifted up mine eyes unto heaven, and mine understanding returned unto me, and I blessed the most High, and I praised and honoured him that liveth for ever, whose dominion is an everlasting dominion, and his kingdom is from generation to generation" (Dan. 4:34).

In spite of how the king must have looked after his long period of living as a beast of the field, his humility was a spiritual revelation! For the first time in his life, he really understood who the one true God of the universe was, as well as the lowly, simple place he occupied as a mere mortal man on this earth. Physically and mentally he must have felt wonderful. He didn't realize just how putrid and befouled he had become from his lifetime of laxity and indulgence. The very king of Babylon was literally "called out of Babylon" by God, an example that would bear much fruit for us, especially those of us "upon whom the ends of the world are come" (1 Cor. 10:11).

Just as with the experiences of the Israelites in the wilderness, let us continue to study and learn from the experiences of those spoken of in the book of Daniel, for the truths contained therein are no longer sealed up but have been opened before us here and now.

Chapter Seven

DUST TO POTTER'S CLAY

To fully understand the significance and the depth of the role that God's heavenly plan for health has for us, it is essential that one have at least a basic understanding of Bible prophecy. This is because prophecy not only shows us the meanings and the purposes of events that have already taken place in history, but it describes with equal clarity things that are yet to come.

As mentioned earlier, the second and seventh chapters of Daniel are closely paralleled, as they describe the same four earthly kingdoms, but in very different ways. Daniel 2 records another dream King Nebuchadnezzar had, which was also interpreted by Daniel. In it a great statue made of four metals was displayed. The head was made of gold, the breast and arms of silver, the belly and thighs of brass, the legs of iron, and finally, the feet of iron mixed with clay. Then a great stone came out of heaven and smashed the statue at its feet, destroying the earthly kingdoms forever and filling the whole earth. Daniel positively identified all the kingdoms described in the king's dream, starting with the statue's head.

"This is the dream; and we will tell the interpretation thereof before the king. Thou, O king ... art this head of gold" (Dan. 2:36–38). So we see here that Babylon was to be the "head of gold" shown in the image.

And then Daniel describes the following kingdoms: "And after thee shall arise another kingdom inferior to thee" (verse 39). This kingdom was represented in the image as the "breast and arms of silver," even as silver is inferior to gold. This kingdom was to be Medo-Persia, as shown in both the Bible and historical records.

And then "another third kingdom of brass, which shall bear rule over all the earth" was to rise up and overtake the Medio-Persian Empire, which was to be ancient Greece. Then was to be the most powerful of them all, the fourth kingdom, which was represented by legs of iron. This was the mighty empire of ancient Rome. It is thus described: "And the fourth kingdom shall be as strong as iron: forasmuch as iron breaketh in pieces and subdueth all things" (verse 40).

Now what are we told regarding the last part of the statue, the feet and toes made partly from iron and part from potter's clay? "And whereas thou sawest the feet and toes, part of potters' clay, and part of iron, the kingdom shall be divided; but there shall be in it of the strength of the iron, forasmuch as thou sawest the iron mixed with miry clay. And as the toes of the feet were part of iron, and part of clay, so the kingdom shall be partly strong, and partly broken. And whereas thou sawest iron mixed with miry clay, they shall mingle themselves with the seed of men: but they shall not cleave one to another, even as iron is not mixed with clay" (verse 41–43).

So, using good old comparative analysis, the most dependable way to understand Scripture, especially symbolic prophecies, what do we know of the feet and toes of the image? We know that it is partly made of the very elements of the ancient Roman Empire, both in form and function. But it shall lack Rome's strength, because it is mixed with clay, and iron and clay do not mix. So what does Scripture tell us about potter's clay? "But now, O Lord, thou art our father; we are the clay, and thou our potter: and we are all the work of thy hand" (Isa. 64:8). And from Paul: "Nay but, O man, who art thou that repliest against God? Shall the thing formed say to him that formed it, Why hast thou made me thus? Hath not the potter power over the clay … ?" (Rom. 9:20, 21).

We, the people of God, are His clay according to Scripture. After all, were we not made "of the dust of the ground" in Eden?

Now why is it that iron and clay cannot mix? Because earthly governments cannot work in harmony with God's kingdom, and the last great world kingdom that shall be smashed to pieces by the great stone that comes forth from heaven will be the result of a human attempt to establish a theocracy unto itself, ruling with the iron hand of Rome while making false pretenses of having the authority of God on earth! God's government on this earth is spiritual. That is what it always has been and always will be.

Only through Christ can you be made a member of God's heavenly kingdom. No earthly powers can ever aid you in receiving that citizenship. Thus we are shown the final end of all earthly kingdoms and the final establishment of God's heavenly kingdom upon the earth: "Thou sawest till that a stone was cut out without hands, which smote the image upon his feet that were of iron and clay, and brake them to pieces. Then was the iron, the clay, the brass, the silver, and the gold, broken to pieces together, and became like the chaff of the summer threshingfloors; and the wind carried them away, that no place was found for them: and the stone that smote the image became a great mountain, and filled the whole earth.... And in the days of these kings shall the God of heaven set up a kingdom, which shall never be destroyed: and the kingdom shall not be left to other people, but it shall break in pieces and consume all these kingdoms, and it shall stand for ever" (Dan. 2:34, 35, 44).

Daniel 7 shows us the same kingdoms as in chapter 2 but with much more detail. This time, instead of the metals on the statue, the kingdoms are represented as four great beasts coming out of the sea (Dan. 7:17), the sea being populated regions as we mentioned before (Rev. 17:15). We know that the first beast, which was "like a lion, and had eagle's wings," was ancient Babylon, which destroyed Jerusalem and the temple and took Daniel and his companions captive to Babylon (Dan. 7:4).

The next two beasts, shown chronologically in order like the metals on the image, were Medo-Persia, shown as a bear with three ribs in its mouth, and ancient Greece, shown as a leopard with four wings and four heads. But it was the last of the great beasts that particularly caught Daniel's attention in his dream: "After this I saw in the night visions, and beheld a fourth beast, dreadful and terrible, and strong exceedingly; and it had great iron teeth: it devoured and brake in pieces, and stamped the residue with the feet of it: and it was diverse from all the beasts that were before it; and it had ten horns" (verse 7). We know that chronologically, this fourth beast has to be the kingdom of Rome, which immediately followed Grecian rule, and it also "had great iron teeth" like the "legs of iron" in the statue. Just as iron is the strongest of metals, it had the power to break and subdue all things before it as depicted by the teeth.

But what particularly troubled Daniel the most about this last kingdom was the blasphemous power that would spring forth from it in the latter days. This other power, though seemingly weaker than the Roman Empire itself, is the same as the feet of the image that was "iron mixed with clay" and in Daniel's dream is called the "little horn," as shown here: "I considered the horns, and, behold, there came up among them another little horn ... and, behold, in this horn were eyes like the eyes of man, and a mouth speaking great things. I beheld, and the same horn made war with the saints, and prevailed against them; ... And he shall speak great words against the most High, and shall wear out the saints of the most High, and think to change times and laws" (verses 8, 21, 25).

So this final power that prevails over the world until the end of time not only comes forth from Rome but is actually Roman by nature, and although it appears not to be powerful in itself, it carries the political influence from its false theocratic rule. Not only this, but it makes "war with the saints" and speaks blasphemous words against the Most High God, actually thinking it has the divine authority to "change times and laws" that God has set for His people to follow.

But, just as with the great stone that came forth from heaven to establish itself, the judgment speaks of the final end of the fourth great beast and the blasphemous little horn power that springs up from it and rules the earth until the final end. "But the judgment shall sit, and they shall take away his dominion, to consume and to destroy it unto the end. And the kingdom and dominion, and the greatness of the kingdom under the whole heaven, shall be given to the people of the saints of the most High, whose kingdom is an everlasting kingdom, and all dominions shall serve and obey him" (verses 6, 27).

Some may wonder if this last-days worldwide rulership that falsely claims to have divine authority is the same power mentioned in Revelation that enforces its mark everywhere with the penalty of a death sentence upon all who do not receive it. To answer that question, let us look at the very roots of why this evil worldwide empire even exists. It began out of the desire to have a kingdom on earth apart from the kingdom of God, and the source of this desire is pure pride, nothing else. So where did pride begin?

Read Isaiah 14:12–16: "How art thou fallen from heaven, O Lucifer, son of the morning! how art thou cut down to the ground, which didst weaken the nations! For thou hast said in thine heart, I will ascend into heaven, I will exalt my throne above the stars of God: I will sit also upon the mount of the congregation, in the sides of the north: I will ascend above the heights of the clouds; I will be like the most High. Yet thou shalt be brought down to hell, to the sides of the pit. They that see thee shall narrowly look upon thee, and consider thee, saying, Is this the man that made the earth to tremble, that did shake kingdoms?"

Shortly after the flood, a community of people desired to protect themselves from any future disasters. They thought they could "build their own tower of safety" to insure that any future punishment from God would not touch them. Secondly they wanted to establish a strong community and avoid being scattered abroad across the earth. But God put an end to the work on the Tower of Babel by confusing their language, thus resulting in the wide variety of languages we have on the earth today. It was here, from a source of confusion and rebellion against God, that the ancient kingdom of Babylon sprang forth, and later served the purpose of bringing severe punishment upon the people of Israel when they refused to keep His commandments and His laws.

Let us now look upon the beast that in the last days attempts to enforce its deadly mark: "And I stood upon the sand of the sea, and saw a beast rise up out of the sea, having seven heads and ten horns, and upon his horns ten crowns, and upon his heads the name of blasphemy. And the beast which I saw was like unto a leopard, and his feet were as the feet of a bear, and his mouth as the mouth of a lion: and the dragon gave him his power, and his seat, and great authority" (Rev. 13:1, 2). Does this beast sound familiar? It should, as it is a conglomeration of all the beasts mentioned in Daniel 7. It has "the mouth of a lion" (Babylon), "the feet of a bear" (Medo-Persia), it is "like unto a leopard" (Greece), it rises "up out of the sea" having "ten horns" (Rome), and it has "upon his heads the name of blasphemy" (the "little horn").

So we see here without question that the modern-day antichrist, which will fully exercise its power in the near future, is simply a continuation of all the world kingdoms from the past that have attempted to rule the world from their own power and authority. The big difference with the antichrist compared to all the past pagan kingdoms is that it will subtly exercise its authority by convincing the world that it is God's representative on earth, when in fact, it is paganism labeled with a Christian name! After all, the beast does not receive its authority from Christ, but from the "dragon," which Scripture identifies as "the great dragon ... that old serpent, called the Devil, and Satan, which deceiveth the whole world" (Rev. 12:9).

But what is the "mark of the beast"? It is the opposite of the seal of God. God's seal, established at Creation and placed at the heart of His law, identifies Him as our one and only Creator. It is for this reason that the seventh-day Sabbath was given to us to eternally remind us that He made us and that He is the source of our life and our existence. The mark of the beast, however, is founded upon blasphemy. It is a false sabbath, having its roots in ancient sun worship, while claiming, without any biblical authority, that it is based upon the resurrection of our Lord on the first day of the week. There is nothing in Scripture, or even in historical records around the time of the early Christian church, suggesting that the seventh-day Sabbath was transferred to the first day of the week. This attempt to change the Sabbath was brought about centuries after the last book of the Bible was written, as an attempt of the Roman Catholic Church to gain political authority through spiritual compromises.

For more information on Bible prophecy and other important biblical topics, I recommend you visit TEACHServices.com or AdventistBookCenter.com.

Chapter Eight

"HE MUST INCREASE"

We are now looking into a time period where the nation of Israel was under Roman rule. The previous kingdoms of Babylon, Medo-Persia and Greece had passed on. The first advent of the Messiah was imminent. Centuries before, Israel was given the exact date of Christ's coming and His crucifixion on the cross, all in the ninth chapter of the book of Daniel, which reads as follows: "Seventy weeks are determined upon thy people and upon thy holy city, to finish the transgression, and to make an end of sins, and to make reconciliation for iniquity, and to bring in everlasting righteousness, and to seal up the vision and prophecy, and to anoint the most Holy. Know therefore and understand, that from the going forth of the commandment to restore and to build Jerusalem unto Messiah the Prince shall be seven weeks, and threescore and two weeks: the street shall be built again, and the wall, even in troublous times.

"And after threescore and two weeks shall Messiah be cut off, but not for himself: and the people of the prince that shall come shall destroy the city and the sanctuary; and the end thereof shall be with a flood, and unto the end of the war desolations are determined. And he shall confirm the covenant with many for one week: and in the midst of the week he shall cause the sacrifice and the oblation to cease, and for the overspreading of abominations he shall make it desolate, even until the consummation, and that determined shall be poured upon the desolate" (Dan. 9:24–27).

This prophecy of the first advent of Christ was written more than five centuries before the event and was predicted far too accurately to be of human design. First, since all Bible prophecy is symbolic (as we have seen before with "beasts" coming out of "seas"), it is also known that a prophetic day in the Bible stands for one year (see Num. 14:34 and Eze. 4:6). Therefore, the "seventy weeks" heretofore mentioned, or 490 days, is actually, in prophetic understanding, 490 years of actual time.

This time period of 490 years, according to the prophecy, was to begin with "the going forth of the commandment to restore and to build Jerusalem unto the Messiah the Prince," which is historically shown to be when the decree of Artaxerxes was given to restore autonomy to the Jewish government (although subject to Persian overlordship). This decree took place in 457 BC.

According to Daniel, this period of probation given to the Israelite nation was to be a time of preparing themselves spiritually for the coming of the Messiah. Nothing more, nothing less. Even the exact dates were given. Christ quoted from these texts when he told His disciples what to watch for in the very last days. He said, "When ye therefore shall see the abomination of desolation, spoken of by Daniel the prophet, stand in the holy place, (whoso readeth, let him understand:) Then let them which be in Judea flee into the mountains: ... But pray ye that your flight be not in the winter, neither on the sabbath day: For then shall be great tribulation, such as was not since the beginning of the world to this time, no, nor ever shall be" (Matt. 24:15–21).

Jesus was to begin His ministry here on earth with a single event, an event that directly preceded His forty-day fast in the wilderness. He was to be baptized by John the Baptist. Let us read of this event. "Then cometh Jesus from Galilee to Jordan unto John, to be baptized of him. But John forbad him, saying, I have need to be baptized of thee, and comest thou to me? And Jesus answering said unto him, Suffer it to be so now: for thus it becometh us to fulfil all righteousness. Then he suffered him. And Jesus, when he was baptized, went up straightway out of the water: and, lo, the heavens were opened unto him, and he saw the Spirit of God descending like a dove, and lighting upon him: And lo a voice from heaven, saying, This is my beloved Son, in whom I am well pleased" (Matt. 3:13–17).

According to all biblical and available historical evidence, Jesus' baptism by John the Baptist took place in AD 27, which was exactly 483 years after the decree of Artaxerxes in 457 BC, which fits perfectly with the "seven weeks, and threescore and two weeks" (69 weeks/483 days), after which "shall Messiah be cut off [killed], but not for himself." Doubts and denial are only for those who are looking for it.

Though comparatively little is written about John the Baptist in Scripture, he played an extremely important role in God's plan, and we have much to learn from his life and ministry. He was literally "the voice of one crying in the wilderness, Prepare ye the way of the Lord, make his paths straight" (Matt. 3:3). He was the one who gave the final warning message that the Messiah was about to come. He was the "Elijah message" that was to precede Christ's first coming and would parallel the same message that will be given by God's faithful followers before His second coming.

We are now living in that time of the second Elijah message. So what did Jesus say of John? "And as they departed, Jesus began to say unto the multitudes concerning John, What went ye out into the wilderness to see? A reed shaken with the wind? But what went ye out for to see? A man clothed in soft raiment? behold, they that wear soft clothing are in kings' houses. But what went ye out for to see? A prophet? yea, I say unto you, and more than a prophet. For this is he, of whom it is written, Behold, I send my messenger before thy face, which shall prepare thy way before thee. Verily I say unto you, Among them that are born of women there hath not risen a greater than John the Baptist: notwithstanding he that is least in the kingdom of heaven is greater than he.

And from the days of John the Baptist until now the kingdom of heaven suffereth violence, and the violent take it by force. For all the prophets and the law prophesied until John. And if ye will receive it, this is Elias [or Elijah], which was for to come. He that hath ears to hear, let him hear" (Matt. 11:7–15).

Jesus recognized John as a prophet and more, saying of him, "among them that are born of women there hath not risen a greater than John the Baptist." Very high recognition and exalted status from the King of kings indeed Yet still, when John was questioned about exactly who he was, he denied being Elijah, or even that he was a prophet at all. Through his humble spirit John showed us that we are to avoid bringing glory and attention to ourselves. John lived a simple and abstemious life. His dress was simple, "his raiment of camel's hair, and a leathern girdle about his loins" was just the opposite of all the self-decoration we see today, and his diet was purely vegetarian, consisting of beans of the locust tree along with wild honey (Matt. 3:4).

John's life was truly an example for those of us in the last days of earth's history to follow. As we near the end of all things, our attitude about how we stand in relation to Christ must be the same as John's when he spoke, "He must increase, but I must decrease" (John 3:30). This shows a level of commitment that is not common in today's world. Yet, we truly have nothing to lose by giving all to Christ, as there is nothing in ourselves, nor in the world we live in, that is really worth hanging onto.

We are now in a time of great enlightenment in earth's history. While our understanding of natural and spiritual law is far behind those who lived during the antediluvian age, God has set this time in earth's history, the last days before Christ's second coming, to be a time when knowledge and understanding of all kinds "shall be increased" significantly beyond that of comparable eras in the world's history.

Today, knowledge of good and evil is increasing. When God reveals light and truth, Satan attempts to counter it with darkness and lies, and whenever and wherever Satan's deceptions seem to dominate, God brings in rays of truth to be received by those who will receive it. The great controversy between Christ and Satan is taking place as never seen before right in front of our eyes.

There are some very notable events that, according to Bible prophecy, had to take place in order for this time of enlightenment to begin. Let us briefly examine some of these events.

First, it was determined that the antichrist, which would come directly out of Rome, would rise to political rulership for an exact amount of time, from the sixth century AD to the eighteenth century AD. This exact time of the rule of the "little horn" is shown as "a time" (one year), "and times" (two years) and "the dividing of time" (one-half a year), or three and a half years, which is also the exact same length as the "forty and two months" that the beast in Revelation 13 was given power. Furthermore, it is also the same amount of time that the church of Christ, when fleeing from Satan, would take shelter in the wilderness—"a thousand two hundred and threescore days." These prophetic times are outlined in Daniel 7:25 and Revelation 12:6 and 13:5.

This is a period of 1260 prophetic days, which is 1260 actual years. During this period of time, known historically as the Dark Ages, knowledge of health and spirituality reached an all time low. Never before had disease of the body, the mind, and the spirit been seen this dramatically for such an extended period of time. While people everywhere were needlessly dying of horrible diseases almost entirely because of a lack of sanitation and malnutrition, people were kept equally in spiritual darkness as the Bible was only read by a select educated few, by those who had been taught the dead language of the ancient Roman Empire. The Scriptures were not generally available in those times to the common person in the spoken languages of their day and time.

Burning stacks of Bibles in prominent public places was often done by this false theocratic power in order to emphasize their power and authority in all matters. It was the teaching then that since the average person did not have the education and spiritual authority to properly interpret and understand the Scriptures that they must be kept "safe" from it for their "own good." Anyone who dared openly defy the unquestioned authority of the church would often be imprisoned and even brutally tortured in the most horrible ways. This was all done by the ruling church authorities in order to "purge" the dissident of any "devils" they may have in them bringing on their rebellious spirit. If after the time spent locked up in dark cells and brutally tortured, they would still refuse to "repent" then they were often publicly put to death by being burned at the stake.

Satan thrives on human ignorance as it helps to serve his purposes in every way. However, before the rule of this great beast, which lasted more than a dozen centuries, came to its end, a new movement was to spring forth, showing the first beams of the shining light of God's Word to the masses. It was known as the great Protestant Reformation. This movement, while protesting the outright evils of the ruling church, sought also to instigate a reform based upon sola scriptura, that is, "by Scripture alone." Just as when God brought Israel out of Egypt, He had to begin His reform on Scripture alone. All true enlightenment is based upon this knowledge.

Many great men of God participated in this movement, which lasted for centuries. One thing the reformers helped to do was bring translations of the Bible to the common person. For example, the King James Version of the Bible was translated in AD 1611 and, to date, has sold billions of copies. Churches were also founded, not upon the authority of the doctrines of people, but upon the Word of God alone.

After the Protestant Reformation had ceased to be a small rebellious movement but had actually become a great power, then the great beast received its "deadly wound," and its perceived absolute spiritual and political power on this earth was broken, but only for a while (Rev. 13:3). Just as the power of the great ruling blasphemous beast was losing its grip on its power, a new nation rose up in a new land, a nation that was founded upon the moral principles of Protestantism and freedom of religion. Its government was "by the people and for the people" instead of operating as a ruling empire, as shown by past kingdoms.

Revelation tells us of this nation. "And I beheld another beast coming up out of the earth; and he had two horns like a lamb, and he spake as a dragon" (Rev. 13:11). So what are we told here? It is a "beast coming up out of the earth." Up to this point in Bible prophecy, all beasts came up out of the sea. So being that we know that a beast coming up out of the sea is a powerful kingdom that comes out of a highly populated region, then the "earth" must refer to the opposite of the sea, that is, a relatively unpopulated region. So we can deduce here that this great kingdom came out of a "new land" where there were no great cities, populations, and kingdoms.

This beast is separate and distinct in this point and in other ways. This new beast also had "two horns like a lamb." We know from Daniel that horns coming out of a beast represent other powers, as it says, "And the ten horns out of this kingdom are ten kings that shall arise" (Dan. 7:24). Yet while the antichrist unsuccessfully attempts to bring these powers together by its own might and strength (the iron and clay of Daniel 2), this new kingdom keeps them apart. We see this in the founding documents of this nation when it guarantees the separation of church and state.

Republicanism and Protestantism are the founding principles of this nation. But since there is no true theocracy upon the earth today, these principles must be kept fundamentally apart. But as long as they are respected and followed by its citizens, the United States of America will thus receive the highest blessing that an earthly kingdom can receive from God. Both the beginning of this new, blessed nation and the temporary end of the power of the great beast took place in the latter part of the eighteenth century. There are no coincidences in God's universe.

However, we also know that before the end of the world and the second coming of Christ this new beast that comes from the land will eventually join with the first beast and enforce its power. As it says, "And he spake as a dragon. And he exerciseth all the power of the first beast before him, and causeth the earth and them which dwell therein to worship the first beast, whose deadly wound was healed" (Rev. 13:11, 12). But before that happens, this great new nation was to be a safe haven for the reform movement and the final message to the world of Christ's return.

As always, when God wants to bring His people back to their forgotten heritage, He starts with the Creation standard. In the early nineteenth century when America was still a bright and shining new nation, the Lord began a movement of health reform. This was sorely needed as in those days knowledge of health and nutrition was not much beyond what they had in the Dark Ages. Just as with the manna in the wilderness, God wanted to lead His people back to His original principles of health in order to prepare them to enter into the Promised Land.

One might even say that the "Moses" of this movement was a Presbyterian minister by the name of Sylvester Graham. This man had found through a lifetime of reading the Scriptures and observing nature, and comparing his personal experiences to those of others, that the original diet God gave humanity at the beginning of Creation was indeed the ideal way of eating, even though people, since then, had strayed far from that ideal. He concluded that if these ideals, found in both the Word of God and in nature, would be followed fully nearly all disease and affliction would virtually disappear. After lengthy periods of time spent in prayerful study and observation, he was ready to make these wonderful truths known to the rest of the world! Why should there be so much unnecessary suffering and sickness?

As such, Graham began a crusade across the nation, showing that God is concerned about our physical health as well as our spiritual health and that the formula for achieving this was very simple and already laid out fully by God for all to see. As John the apostle says, "Beloved, I wish above all things that thou mayest prosper and be in health, even as thy soul prospereth" (3 John 2).

Graham emphasized a life based upon biblical moral principles and abstemious living habits and that any type of overindulgence would lead to downfall, both physically and spiritually. Also, as a rebuke to the widespread use of refined grain products during his day, he invented a whole-grain cracker, which to this day, is known by his name as "graham crackers."

A young follower of Graham who was greatly inspired by his work and teachings was John Harvey Kellogg. And yes, he invented the famous corn flakes we know also by his name today. But actually, it was his brother, Will, who wanted to market and mass-produce them, as Dr. John Kellogg had originally designed them to be used for his patients at the Battle Creek Sanitarium in Battle Creek, Michigan. The sanitarium at Battle Creek was an amazing center of health and healing. The treatments at the facility were based upon the principles of nature and Scripture.

These men accomplished a widespread influence for good. Yet, however wonderful the knowledge of health is, we must never forget that we are only mortal beings, we are but dust. "And the Lord God formed man of the dust of the ground, and breathed into his nostrils the breath of life; and man became a living soul" (Gen. 2:7). And when this creative process is reversed at death, the psalmist tells us that "his breath goeth forth, he returneth to his earth; in that very day his thoughts perish" (Ps. 146:4).

It is, therefore, logical that since our "thoughts perish" and we cease to exist after death we must ask God what hope we have. What lies beyond this life? The Bible makes it clear that Jesus died for our sins, was raised from the grave and returned to heaven to live with God the Father and the angels; thus, we can have faith that we also will be raised up into eternal life. Paul, in speaking on this subject, wrote to the Thessalonicans, "But I would not have you to be ignorant, brethren, concerning them which are asleep [dead], that ye sorrow not, even as others which have no hope. For if we believe that Jesus died and rose again, even so them also which sleep in Jesus will God bring with him. For this we say unto you by the word of the Lord, that we which are alive and remain unto the coming of the Lord shall not prevent them which are asleep" (1 Thess. 4:13–15).

And what amazing event takes place as the righteous dead are being raised to life? "For the Lord himself shall descend from heaven with a shout, with the voice of the archangel, and with the trump of God: and the dead in Christ shall rise first: Then we which are alive and remain shall be caught up together with them in the clouds, to meet the Lord in the air: and so shall we ever be with the Lord. Wherefore comfort one another with these words" (verses 16–18). Our hope beyond this life resides in one event, the second coming of our Lord and Savior Jesus Christ. At this time He Himself will call forth the dead from their graves, and all the problems that plagued us in the past will become just that, a thing of the past.

Paul describes this again to the believers in Corinth. "Behold, I shew you a mystery; We shall not all sleep, but we shall all be changed, In a moment, in the twinkling of an eye, at the last trump: for the trumpet shall sound, and the dead shall be raised incorruptible, and we shall be changed. For this corruptible must put on incorruption, and this mortal must put on immortality. So when this corruptible shall have put on incorruption, and this mortal shall have put on immortality, then shall be brought to pass the saying that is written, Death is swallowed up in victory" (1 Cor. 15:51–54).

Therefore, just as God was reminding people of the forgotten knowledge of His health principles, He also inspired another movement that would parallel the revival in understanding of health and hygiene. This was known as the Second Advent movement of the mid-nineteenth century. This increase in knowledge regarding the coming of our Lord to claim His own was truly the consummation of what the Lord had done to release His people from the Dark Ages that had shrouded them from understanding, to a time of increased knowledge that began with the Protestant Reformation, which then continued with the birth of a new nation that would be the ideal breeding ground for the bringing forth of the sacred and eternal truths He wanted to reveal to the entire world.

The leader of this movement to proclaim the second coming of the Messiah was a Baptist minister named William Miller.

Though this great and wonderful movement served to bring to the attention of everyone the importance of the second advent of Christ in the plan of salvation, there was a fatal flaw in his interpretation of last-day Bible prophecy. While Miller had the prophetic dates accurately predicted, it was his understanding of the events that would take place at the appointed time that caused his theory to come crashing down.

Like so many other Christians, Miller had placed great hope in the second coming of the Lord. He was waiting for that great and wonderful day of promise that is the hope of every son and daughter of Christ. Miller had been studying the prophecies of the end times, particularly those of Daniel and Revelation, for many years and had reached the inescapable conclusion that the cleansing of the sanctuary (Dan. 8:14) would take place 2300 years after the decree of Artaxerxes in 457 BC, and would thus reach its fulfillment in the middle of the nineteenth century. However, his great error in interpretation was in assuming that the "sanctuary" thus mentioned was the earth itself, and that its "cleansing" was to be that of the cleansing of the earth by fire at the second coming of Christ (2 Peter 3:6, 7).

As a result, Miller believed and taught adamantly for many years leading up to the appointed date in Daniel 8 that Christ would be returning and the righteous dead would be resurrected and the world would be destroyed. However, when this prophetic date came and went uneventfully, both Miller and his many steadfast followers were disappointed and heartbroken beyond imagination. This time in history is known as the Great Disappointment. Yet in spite of all the negative feelings that surrounded this event, an interest in Christ's second coming such as had never been seen before in the Protestant movement sprang forth.

The mistake that Miller made was in setting an exact date for the coming of Christ. Of this, Jesus said, "But of that day and hour knoweth no man, no, not the angels in heaven, but my Father only. But as the days of Noe were, so shall also the coming of the Son of man be. For as in the days that were before the flood they were eating and drinking, marrying and giving in marriage, until the day that Noe entered into the ark, And knew not until the flood came, and took them all away; so shall also the coming of the Son of man be" (Matt. 24:36–39).

So, not only is it impossible for anyone to know the exact date of Christ's coming, but Miller's other main error was in his understanding of just what the sanctuary was in Daniel 8:14. The only way to interpret Scripture without error is by comparatively analyzing everything that is said on the subject that is being studied, and to study it in its context (Isa. 28:10).

In the book of Hebrews we are told that Christ is our High Priest in heaven. "We have such an high priest, who is set on the right hand of the throne of the Majesty in the heavens; A minister of the sanctuary, and of the true tabernacle, which the Lord pitched, and not man" (Heb. 8:1, 2). We should also consider the words of Isaiah the prophet regarding this matter. "Thus saith the Lord, The heaven is my throne, and the earth is my footstool: where is the house that ye build unto me? and where is the place of my rest?" (Isa. 66:1).

So we see plainly written in Scripture that while the earth is the Lord's "footstool" it is definitely not His throne, nor His sanctuary. We know from Scripture that the true sanctuary, the Lord's temple where He presently dwells, is in heaven, not on earth! The earthly temple that Moses built was only a copy, a "shadow of heavenly things, as Moses was admonished of God when he was about to make the tabernacle," of which God gave him a pattern to use as the design, "See, saith he, that thou make all things according to the pattern shewed to thee in the mount" (Heb. 8:5). This "pattern" was to show us, in form and function, the very plan of salvation itself and the heavenly model. There is even an ark of the covenant containing the original Ten Commandments in the Most Holy Place of the heavenly sanctuary!

John the apostle saw and described the heavenly sanctuary in vision: "And the temple of God was opened in heaven, and there was seen in his temple the ark of his testament" (Rev. 11:19). And again in Hebrews is says, "Neither by the blood of goats and calves, but by his own blood he entered in once into the holy place, having obtained eternal redemption for us.... For Christ is not entered into the holy places made with hands, which are the figures of the true; but into heaven itself, now to appear in the presence of God for us" (Heb. 9:12, 24).

Regarding the earthly temple given through Moses, its final purpose and place ended at the cross of Christ. The sacrifices and offerings were no longer necessary to be offered at a temple made with human hands. It was no longer necessary for a sinful, mortal priest to stand between God and the people. Now we have a far better High Priest. Having obtained eternal redemption for us, Jesus stands before the Father in the heavenly temple. The end of the place and purpose of the earthly temple was shown when Christ died on the cross. "Jesus, when he had cried again with a loud voice, yielded up the ghost. And, behold, the veil of the temple was rent in twain from the top to the bottom; and the earth did quake, and the rocks rent" (Matt. 27:50, 51).

Not only was the reason for the existence of an earthly sanctuary completely eliminated on the cross, but Christ also predicted its total destruction in the future. "And Jesus went out, and departed from the temple: and his disciples came to him for to shew him the buildings of the temple. And Jesus said unto them, See ye not all these things? verily I say unto you, There shall not be left here one stone upon another, that shall not be thrown down" (Matt. 24:1, 2).

Returning to Miller's prediction regarding the cleansing of the sanctuary, the date was right, and it was clear that a cleansing would indeed take place, but it can be deduced that it involved the heavenly sanctuary and not anything on this earth. We know for sure this was to be an event central to the plan of salvation and that it would take place just before the coming of Christ, yet we would not see it with our very own eyes. We know that chronologically it would take place after the birth of the new nation that came out of the earth with horns like a lamb, just after the antichrist little horn would have its power taken away, allowing a revival to take place in this land that would feed the earth with its truths.

This unseen event was to take place in heaven itself, and it is the final judgment of all God's people upon the earth, both alive and dead. Daniel records this event just after the little horn's power is taken away. "I beheld till thrones were cast down, and the Ancient of days did sit, whose garment was white as snow, and the hair of his head like the pure wool: his throne was like the fiery flame, and his wheels as burning fire. A fiery stream issued and came forth from before him: thousand thousands ministered unto him, and ten thousand times ten thousand stood before him: the judgment was set, and the books were opened" (Dan. 7:9, 10).

Before Christ can come and complete the total plan of our salvation, which is the resurrection of the righteous dead and the transformation and eternal glorification of all of God's saints, the final judgment of all of the redeemed in Christ must be laid open for the universe to see. (Yes, there are other populated, unfallen worlds throughout God's vast creation. We are not the only ones.) During the cleansing of the sanctuary is when the books were opened. A cursory look at Revelation 20:1–4 reveals another investigative judgment that takes place. This is the judgment of the wicked. It takes place during the thousand years after Christ's coming, and even though the books will be opened here as well, there will be no cleansing of the sanctuary as with the judgment of the righteous.

The cleansing of the sanctuary in heaven is actually done with the blood of Christ Himself, carried into the heavenly sanctuary before God the Father just as the earthly priests did once a year on a Jewish holy day called the Day of Atonement. On this holiest of all the ceremonial Sabbaths, the high priest would enter into the Holy of Holies, the place where the ark of the covenant resided, and sprinkle the blood of the animal sacrifice, symbolizing the purging of all the sins of Israel forever from the record books of heaven. Christ was slain as our Passover Lamb when He died on the cross, but now He stands in the heavenly temple before God the Father, ministering as our High Priest above.

Although all the ceremonial holy days (see Lev. 23) ended at the cross, as they were based upon the earthly temple services, we can still learn much from studying these lessons as they were all given by God to Israel to teach them His plan of salvation for them, and we, too, can learn the same. (Note also that the prophecies regarding the Messiah and the heavenly sanctuary in Daniel 8 and 9 closely complement the descriptions given in Hebrews 8 and 9.)

We are now in a day and time in earth's history when all that was previously hidden is now being made known. We can claim all the knowledge and wisdom that our forefathers who wrote the Scriptures did not fully see. The seals that shut Daniel have been opened, revealing these truths. Covering our eyes will not prevent the light from shining forth. And if we don't understand, Christ is ready and willing to "anoint thine eyes with eyesalve, that thou mayest see" (Rev. 3:18).

Chapter Ten

HIS OTHER TEMPLE

We have just seen how important the cleansing of the heavenly temple is to God's plan of salvation, but God has another temple. It is on this earth. It is us, our bodies. "Know ye not that ye are the temple of God, and that the Spirit of God dwelleth in you? If any man defile the temple of God, him shall God destroy; for the temple of God is holy, which temple ye are" (1 Cor. 3:16, 17). And Paul, when writing to the Corinthians, emphasizes this point a second time: "What? know ye not that your body is the temple of the Holy Ghost which is in you, which ye have of God, and ye are not your own? For ye are bought with a price: therefore glorify God in your body, and in your spirit, which are God's" (1 Cor. 6:19, 20).

In these last days of earth's history, the record books in heaven are being cleansed of our sins forever, for all eternity. But in order for this to actually take place, God's other temple on earth—us— the one where His Holy Spirit presently resides, must be correspondingly cleansed as well. For this to be, God must return His people back to the original standard He gave them at the creation of the world. We cannot linger in the past, using the mistakes of those that preceded us as excuses. If God is to restore His own back to His image before the end of all things comes upon us, we must remember the three points of God's Creation standard: 1) the seventh-day Sabbath, 2) the sanctity of marriage, and 3) the original diet.

God wanted His people, the children of Israel, to follow these before they entered the Promised Land, but because of their resistance, He could only make the Sabbath an absolute as written in the Ten Commandments. They rejected the ideal diet, as clearly shown in the test of the manna and the quail. And the true nature of what marriage really stood for could not be fully revealed until the first advent of Christ, as the Bridegroom (Christ) was introduced to the bride (His church).

We are now under the microscope of the universe. Every eye in the heavens looks upon us with discernment as to whether or not we shall choose to serve Christ or Satan. We are no longer living in the times of ignorance, which God "winked at." Everything is being fully revealed before all, and God "now commandeth all men every where to repent" (Acts 17:30).

The latter rain of the Holy Spirit is upon us, as spoken of by the prophet Joel. "And it shall come to pass afterward, that I will pour out my spirit upon all flesh; and your sons and your daughters shall prophesy, your old men shall dream dreams, your young men shall see visions: And also upon the servants and upon the handmaids in those days will I pour out my spirit. And I will shew wonders in the heavens and in the earth, blood, and fire, and pillars of smoke. The sun shall be turned into darkness, and the moon into blood, before the great and terrible day of the Lord come. And it shall come to pass, that whosoever shall call on the name of the Lord shall be delivered: for in mount Zion and in Jerusalem shall be deliverance, as the Lord hath said, and in the remnant whom the Lord shall call" (Joel 2:28–32).

This prophecy received partial fulfillment in Acts 2, being that it was the "former rain moderately" (Joel 2:23), which took place in only a small part of the world, that is, Jerusalem, but when the latter rain comes, it shall be a worldwide event. During these times, the Lord will call a remnant to stand strong for Him. So who is this remnant, and what identifies them? Turn to Revelation 12:17: "And the dragon was wroth with the woman [Christ's church], and went to make war with the remnant of her seed, which keep the commandments of God, and have the testimony of Jesus Christ."

The remnant of God's people are said to be those who "keep the commandments of God, and have the testimony of Jesus Christ."

First of all, they keep *all* the commandments of God. Not just some or most of them, but all ten of them. Remember, James said, "For whosoever shall keep the whole law, and yet offend in one point, he is guilty of all" (James 2:10). God's remnant people will also have the "testimony of Jesus Christ." We are told in Scripture, by the word of an angel speaking to John, that "the testimony of Jesus is the spirit of prophecy" (Rev. 19:10). While there are many "gifts of the Spirit" mentioned in Scripture (see 1 Cor. 12), apparently the one spiritual gift that stands out as an identifying mark of God's remnant people in the last days is the gift of prophecy. This is not surprising, as Joel points out its significance in the former and latter rains of the Holy Spirit, and Paul also, in the fourteenth chapter of 1 Corinthians, emphasizes the superiority of prophecy over the other gifts.

It goes without saying that while God's remnant people are seemingly small and unrecognized by many they will have their roots in all the righteous movements of truth that God has raised up to this point in history. The Protestant Reformation, Sylvester Graham's health movement, and William Miller's Second Advent movement are all great "trees of truth" from which God's last-day, commandment-keeping people will have been a part of.

One of the most important truths that God's remnant shall teach the world in the last days is the final reformation to restore God's original Creation plan to His people. The Sabbath was re-established at Mt. Sinai. Marriage was restored during Christ's ministry on earth. But now, as the final judgment of God's saints takes place in heaven and the final message of warning goes to the world to not receive the mark of the beast, we are to fully reveal the original standard that the Lord set up from the foundation of the world.

The "missing link" in the chain of God's original plan is the original diet. It has been swept aside and virtually forgotten by those who claim to be God's people. Why? Because appetite is the original sin, and Satan uses it to subtly creep in and assure us that we can indulge without fear of consequences. He continually tells us as he did Eve, "Ye shall not surely die." Many of Christ's followers are repeating the mistakes of the Israelites in the wilderness.

Instead, we, the faithful few of the Lord, should be as Daniel when he and his friends were captured and taken to Babylon and they refused to defile themselves with the king's food and drink. We need to be as John the Baptist, living an abstinent life from the plant products of the land and proclaiming the Elijah message of the last days. We need to be as Jesus when the devil tempted him in the wilderness, and he said, "If thou be the Son of God, command that these stones be made bread. But he answered and said, It is written, Man shall not live by bread alone, but by every word that proceedeth out of the mouth of God" (Matt. 4:3, 4).

Unfortunately, some have come to the false conclusion that true health is almost totally centered around diet and food, and everything else is of little or no importance. As important as diet is to health, we must look at all aspects of the equation as we examine the important role of overcoming the appetite in the sanctification of Christ's followers in the last days.

Chapter Eleven
GOD'S PRESCRIPTION FOR US

God has a prescription for perfect health. It is written in the laws of nature, very much the same way God wrote His moral law in tablets of stone. We will always receive benefits by following His laws. As with Israel, we gain blessings by obedience and curses from disobedience. So often we tend to complain when these curses befall us, but as we have seen from the beginning of human history, God's curses are really consequences given out of love, as a parent would handle their child.

Following are eight natural remedies: 1) pure air, 2) sunlight, 3) abstemiousness, 4) rest, 5) exercise, 6) proper diet, 7) water, and 8) trust in God. They are based upon fundamental health principles that have their roots in Creation itself, and are the guidelines through which all true health is obtained. To attempt to add or take away any one of these principles would only result in a compromise of one's own personal state of health. It may seem like such a simple formula, but all of God's truths are really basic and easy to understand. People tend to make everything so complicated!

On the following pages we will examine each of the eight natural remedies.

Pure Air

The more we get of this the better! After all, our breathing never stops. We always need a fresh supply of oxygen. The more we are around plants and trees the better, as they not only take in the carbon dioxide that we give off as a waste product, but they give off oxygen we need. Be around plants as much as you can. Unless you live in a highly polluted urban area, being outdoors is always far better than indoors, for many reasons. Get outside!

Sunlight

The sun is essential to all life on earth. We need sunlight. Direct exposure on the skin is essential to good health. While a good tan is usually associated with good health, it can also be a result of obsessive behavior. Overexposure is never healthy. Know your limits. Sunscreen is unnatural. If you know you're going to be in the sun longer than you should, then you need a wide-brimmed hat and some loose, light-colored cotton clothing that covers your skin. Sunbathing can be wonderful, even in the wintertime. If you are light-complected, plant a couple of aloe vera plants. In the event that you accidentally get a little scorched, the soothing gel from the leaves of the plant will assist in a natural recovery.

Abstemiousness

For those not familiar with this word, it is the same as "temperate" and "moderation" in the Bible. "And every man that striveth for the mastery is temperate in all things" (1 Cor. 9:25). And Philippians 4:5 says, "Let your moderation be known unto all men." It is a universal law of health that applies to all the other natural remedies, except for the eighth, for one cannot ever trust too much in God. Otherwise, we can "overdo" and "underdo" practically anything. We should always strive to maintain a balance.

Rest

When God first created the earth, He gave us the "evening and the morning" as separate times of activity and inactivity. Our circadian rhythms are based upon the fact that we are day-dwelling creatures and not nocturnal. No matter how many years one lives their life out of harmony with these natural rhythms, their bodies still recognize the rising and the setting of the sun as the time when they should be awake and active. "Early to bed and early to rise makes a man healthy, wealthy and wise," goes the saying.

At Creation, God also gave us one out of every seven days of the week to rest and to put aside all the cares and worries of life. When properly observed, the Sabbath is truly a blessing that God gave for all mankind to enjoy.

Exercise

This is a natural remedy where we really need to avoid extremes! We so often see people avoiding exercise altogether, and others do just the opposite, making it into an obsession. Is there a place where you can take a walk? Well, then you can start exercising! No need for a gym membership, a pool, or any special equipment people always tell you "you have to have" to start working out. You don't even need any special shoes or clothing. Just get out and start walking every day, or whenever you can. It can be either a laid-back relaxing experience, or you can really make it into a heart-thumping sweaty workout. It's entirely your choice. Don't think of exercise as "all or nothing." With exercise, a little is always better than none at all.

Along with walking, the other exercise that was part of God's original plan was that of gardening, which was Adam's first job in the Garden of Eden. Of course, as the record shows, the work got tougher after the fall, but Adam was still to "till the ground." Walking and working with plants outdoors is God's original exercise plan for us.

Proper Diet

"You are what you eat." Proper diet is pretty important, isn't it? After all, a building is only as strong as the materials you make it from. Everything we need to know about proper diet and our eating habits is found in the Holy Bible and Mother Nature. People's little discoveries really don't tell us anything we need and already haven't been told.

Water

Nature's perfect cleanser, both inside and outside the body. It is second only to the air for our immediate survival needs. The best water is absolutely pure, nothing added, nothing taken away. Get the best drinking water you can. Your health is worth the investment.

Trust in God

This is truly the foundation that all the other natural remedies are built upon. Without this one, all the others will eventually crumble. There are those that make a god unto themselves, thinking they can achieve perfect health in this life, and thereby they devote their entire lives to following the first seven of the eight natural remedies, leaving out the "chief Cornerstone"! What they fail to see is that the whole point and purpose of following God's laws of health is to keep and maintain the best possible "body temple" for the Holy Spirit to occupy while here on this earth.

Of course, we know that perfect health will not be achieved until the second coming of Jesus Christ!

Chapter Twelve
THE SPARK OF LIFE

Life. It is by far the most profound thing God has created in the entire universe. Human beings have theorized and philosophized about it for centuries, but most truly cannot figure it out. So just what is life? Well, we know it is the opposite of death. Life is positive. It is an active force in the creation of God, whereas death is absolute nothingness, a void where life once was but no longer is. A rock is not dead, simply because it was never alive, whereas a totally burnt tree is dead because the life that once resided in it's now charred remains and is gone.

Though we were originally formed by the hand of God from inorganic elements, the dust of the ground, God breathed into us His own personal breath of life, and at that moment Adam became a living soul. All life is formed from these two elements, the dust of the ground and the breath of life. This includes all creatures, whether man or beast, animal or vegetable.

In this world, we are all mortal and subject to death. King Solomon wrote, "For that which befalleth the sons of men befalleth beasts; even one thing befalleth them: as the one dieth, so dieth the other; yea, they have all one breath … All go unto one place; all are of the dust, and all turn to dust again" (Eccl. 3:19, 20). So what is the difference between people and all other created beings? First, we were all made in God's own image, physically, mentally, and spiritually. Second, Christ our Creator became one of us and paid the penalty for our sins by dying on the cross. These things only apply to the human race. While we are to respect and take proper care of God's creation, it is we, the human race, who are the crowning act of God's creation on this earth, and we should never forget this.

In these very last days God is making His final call to humanity. He pleads with us to choose life rather than death. Our obsession with death, when we were designed to be creatures of life, is beyond comprehension. He says to us through Ezekiel the prophet, "Have I any pleasure at all that the wicked should die? saith the Lord God: and not that he should return from his ways and live? ... Yet saith the house of Israel, The way of the Lord is not equal. O house of Israel, are not my ways equal? are not your ways unequal? Therefore I will judge you, O house of Israel, every one according to his ways, saith the Lord God. Repent, and turn yourselves from all your transgressions; so iniquity shall not be your ruin. Cast away from you all your transgressions, whereby ye have transgressed; and make you a new heart and a new spirit: for why will ye die, O house of Israel? For I have no pleasure in the death of him that dieth, saith the Lord God: wherefore turn yourselves, and live ye" (Eze. 18:23–32).

When God first gave Noah and his family the flesh of animals to eat, He gave them an explicit order not to eat the blood of the animal. Why? "For the life of the flesh is in the blood" (Lev. 17:11). Blood is very volatile. It is literally the "river of life" that unceasingly carries oxygen and nutrients to all the cells and tissues of the body while simultaneously taking away the products of waste from the cells, delivering them to the organs of excretion. Once death occurs, the blood immediately begins to become very foul, putrid, and toxic. It should never be eaten. Only a true carnivorous creature, which humans are not, can subsist and thrive eating large quantities of flesh and blood.

Spiritually, on the other hand, it is by eating the flesh and drinking the blood of Christ that we gain salvation. Read John 6:53, 54: "Then Jesus said unto them, Verily, verily, I say unto you, Except ye eat the flesh of the Son of man, and drink his blood, ye have no life in you. Whoso eateth my flesh, and drinketh my blood, hath eternal life; and I will raise him up in the last day."

To have true health we must only have Christ in us. This applies physically as well as spiritually. We are to be a living sacrifice unto our Lord. Paul said to the Romans, "I beseech you therefore, brethren, by the mercies of God, that ye present your bodies a living sacrifice, holy, acceptable unto God, which is your reasonable service. And be not conformed to this world: but be ye transformed by the renewing of your mind, that ye may prove what is that good, and acceptable, and perfect, will of God" (Rom. 12:1, 2).

We know that we cannot really eat the flesh and drink the blood of Christ, so what do we physically consume so that our bodies can be at their best level of health? First and foremost, only eat foods that God created "in the beginning" for us to eat that still have "the spark of life," that is, the "breath of God," in them. We know from Scripture that people are not naturally flesh-eaters. And meat does not have the spark of life still in it when you go to eat it. There is no such thing as "living" flesh-food as the moment the animal is slaughtered, the life force is gone and putrefaction begins to immediately set in. Plants, however, are different in that they can maintain their life force for long periods of time even after being removed from their life-giving environments.

Have you ever seen a seed grow or a potato sprout, even after long periods of being in storage? That is the long stored-up energy of which I speak. Though dormant, it still resides in the plants, which can suddenly spring to life even after years in a dark, cold environment. Basically, we should eat all of our food when it is still alive, so that we may receive the life force God placed in it. After all, why would we want to eat anything that is dead?

This question may seem plain and simple enough, yet it is a fact that human beings today mostly consume food that is dead, and comparatively little of that which is alive. This is the direct result of what I call DFA, "Dead Food Addiction." It is the most widespread and readily accepted of all addictions around the globe, which is according to Satan's plan.

All addictions are a form of obsessive/compulsive behavior, where a person, for any number of reasons, begins to form a habitual cycle that, while it may seem pleasurable, does great harm in the long run. While addictions can be physical or mental, in many cases they are both. It goes without saying that the longer the addiction is indulged, the more deeply ingrained it will be. With DFA, for most people it is literally a life-long habitual way of thinking and behaving passed from one generation to the next with nothing but total approval and encouragement from everyone around them to continue down its deadly path. Alcohol and drug addictions are actually easier to "come clean" from than DFA, because the results of these monstrous habits are far more obvious and are surrounded by disapproval from nearly everyone.

If Adam and Eve had started destroying the life-force within their food immediately after leaving Eden, their lifespan and that of every successive generation would have begun to immediately decline. No matter how otherwise "pure" or "clean" one's food may be, if all its life force has been removed, it is dead! Only by an outright miracle of God, can life spring forth from that which is dead. If we consume death, we automatically bring forth death unto ourselves. It is as plain as day.

People began changing and "processing" their food shortly after the flood, no doubt because of the extreme changes in their daily diet. In order to make eating the animal flesh palatable, it was deemed necessary to season it and mix it with other foods and prepare it in various ways. But the most destructive form of food preparation is to cook it over the fire. The primary purpose of fire is to destroy—it obliterates all life that stands in its way.

Let us look at a few examples of fire in Scripture. "For, behold, the Lord will come with fire, and with his chariots like a whirlwind, to render his anger and fury, and his rebuke with flames of fire.

For by fire and by his sword will the Lord plead with all flesh: and the slain of the Lord shall be many. They that sanctify themselves, and purify themselves in the gardens behind one tree in the midst, eating swine's flesh, and the abomination, and the mouse, shall be consumed together, saith the Lord" (Isa. 66:15–17). Malachi the prophet speaks in this regard: "For, behold, the day cometh, that shall burn as an oven; and all the proud, yea, and all that do wickedly, shall be stubble: and the day that cometh shall burn them up, saith the Lord of hosts, that it shall leave them neither root nor branch.... And ye shall tread down the wicked; for they shall be ashes under the soles of your feet in the day that I shall do this, saith the Lord of hosts" (Mal. 4:1, 3). John, in the book of Revelation, also describes the Lord's final act of purification by the use of fire: "Satan shall be loosed out of his prison, And shall go out to deceive the nations which are in the four quarters of the earth ... And they went up on the breadth of the earth, and compassed the camp of the saints about, and the beloved city: and fire came down from God out of heaven, and devoured them" (Rev. 20:7–9).

Through Scripture and by personal experience, we know that fire destroys life. When people began processing their food with fire, they began to eat that which is dead. An "unfired" seed will sprout and form a new plant, but have you ever tried planting a roasted seed? It will rot away as all the life is gone from it. So it is when we eat dead food. It "rots away" in our insides, bringing forth the symptoms of death. In a "nutshell" (pun intended), God's original and perfect diet that He gave us to live by consisted only of fruits, unripe grains, tender legumes, nuts, and various oily seeds, and then vegetables were added after the fall. All of these were to be eaten in their whole, natural, "unfired" state, with nothing added and nothing taken away. This was the ideal plan for living at the creation of the world, and it remains so to this day. Any attempt to deviate from that complete and perfect plan for living only results in a corresponding downfall in our health.

When God's original diet plan is followed and the old habits and addictions fade into the past, one realizes just how foolish it was to be a virtual slave to one's appetite, which has been perverted by a lifetime of deviations from natural law. An internal sense of balance, a clarity of mind, is reached that you probably previously thought to be unattainable. You may say to yourself, "Wow! Why didn't someone tell me about this before? This is so wonderful!" A sense of harmony with both nature and God is reached that will seem like a dream come true. I am not exaggerating on this point. The only way you can confirm this is to try it for yourself. At first, you may go through some "withdrawals" as you transition from "Egypt" to the "Promised Land," but if you stand fast, they will pass with time. That is where the Israelites failed in the wilderness; they were not patient with the Lord. We must not complain for what we have been denied, but be thankful for what we have. A meek and quiet spirit is the greatest key to achieving success in breaking the Dead Food Addiction and returning to God's original diet.

Inevitably, the question about what Jesus ate while on this earth comes up when we talk about diet and Christian character. Some say, "Well, wasn't Jesus perfect? And didn't He eat fish and bread?" The obvious biblical response to this question is that although the first advent of Jesus was the beginning of the time of reformation, the end and full consummation of that time will not be completed until the final judgment just before the second coming of Christ.

Although Christ restored marriage to its proper place during His ministry on earth, the restoration of the original diet was yet to come. Just as with Moses and the Israelites regarding marriage, so it was not yet time to reveal the full truths of the complete Creation standard. Still, many will doubt this point as they say, "Why should I be any better than Jesus?" To this I will respond, "Because Jesus says so!" If you don't believe me, read this verse: "Verily, verily, I say unto you, He that believeth on me, the works that I do shall he do also; and greater works than these shall he do; because I go unto my Father" (John 14:12).

Jesus Himself said that His followers are to do even "greater works" than He did. Why is this so? "Because I go unto my Father." When Christ left the earth in His glorified form, He promised us that we would receive the full blessings of the Holy Spirit as never been seen before. How was this possible? Because when He came the first time to the earth, it was as a servant, meek and lowly, who was to be slain as the sacrifice for our sins. Now, He is our High Priest in heaven, ministering in the sanctuary above in the very presence of the Father Himself. Now He can pour out the fullness of His knowledge, power, and blessings upon the earth as never been seen! The "ante has been upped" as we near the end of time, and God's people are indeed expected to do "greater works" than even our Lord Himself did when He dwelt among us.

For those who are seeking the truth, the reasons are all there to follow this final reformation of God's people. Human beings and all life on earth are weaker and more degenerated than ever before. Animals and people grow more diseased with the passing of time. The very environment itself is beginning to collapse under the curses caused by humanity, and if for no other cause, the purely physical reasons are enough for returning back to our Creation roots!

Christ stands right now in the Most Holy Place of the heavenly sanctuary judging His own, both the living and dead, from the record books in heaven. The great controversy between Christ and Satan will reach a head in our day as has never been seen before. Everything is being laid open before the universe. If there was ever a time, a time when humanity is at its weakest and the powers of Satan are at their fullest, when we need our physical and mental faculties to be functioning at full capacity, it is now. Instead of repeating the mistakes of the Israelites in the wilderness, let us look to the successes of Daniel when taken captive to Babylon as we prepare for the last days.

Chapter Thirteen

SEASONS, TIMES, AND PURPOSES

We are part of this earth. We are made of the dust of the earth, and we were made to inhabit the earth. Likewise, the finely timed rhythms of our body are distinctly set by the rhythms of the earth. When God made the earth, He gave us night and day: "And God called the light Day, and the darkness he called Night. And the evening and the morning were the first day" (Gen. 1:5).

Humans are naturally tropical/sub-tropical creatures. Had it not been for the fall, people would not have migrated to inhospitable climates. The equatorial ideal is a twelve-hour day that is confirmed in Scripture. "Jesus answered, Are there not twelve hours in the day?" (John 11:9). Basically, people are diurnal, that is, a day creature, instead of nocturnal, one that sleeps during the day and is active at night. Even though we may attempt to defy this with artificial lighting and television, it still remains a constant—humans are creatures of the day, not the night. Our internal clocks are timed to the rising and the setting of the sun. We cannot rework the laws of nature to suit our fancy anymore than the citizens of Babel could build a tower to escape any possible future deluge.

Both our sleep and our digestion are subject to these natural rhythms in our bodies. Even though humanity has settled itself in parts of the world where the days can be very short in the winter, the equatorial and biblical standard of the twelve-hour day is what we should live by, wherever we may happen to be. In Scripture, during the annual solar equinoxes, the "first hour" of the day began at what we would call 6 a.m., the "sixth hour" was at noon, and the day ended at 6 p.m. Our digestion is timed to this schedule.

During the daylight hours, digestion of food works at peak effi-ciency, but at night, it considerably drops off, coming to a virtual halt late in the evening. When food remains in the stomach over-night, it does not digest at all, but rather it literally rots, becoming foul and putrid, and thus poisoning the system. Innumerable di-gestive problems and health problems in general could be avoided if people would not go to bed with food still in their stomachs. Late, heavy suppers and constant snacking are the primary causes of these widespread problems.

To get started on the right foot, begin the day with a good, wholesome breakfast. Fruits are the best energy food we have, and energy is what we need to get us through the day. But nuts and various seeds provide satiety and "hold us down" till the next meal. Fruits should be eaten more liberally, while the nuts and oil-seeds should be used in moderation. It takes about one-half of a biblical "day," that is, about six hours, for the body to not only fully digest and assimilate a meal but to prepare itself to receive another meal. For this reason, eating between meals should be avoided. The wise man, King Solomon wrote, "Eat in due season, for strength, and not for drunkenness!" (Eccl. 10:17), thus show-ing that to not eat in "due season" leads to "drunkenness."

Eating at the wrong times can and will lead to a form of intoxi-cation! It's not just "what" you eat, but "how" you eat that makes a difference. The process of digestion is at its peak early in the morning, and it gradually wanes off as the day moves toward eve-ning, dropping off rapidly after dark. Yet, as important as a good breakfast is, the biggest objection to not having an early breakfast is that people complain of not having any appetite in the morning. Well, when you wake up in the morning with the remnants of a mostly undigested and partially putrid meal in your stomach from the night before, it's easy to see why you wouldn't have an appetite in the morning! The key to not being ravenously hungry throughout the day and evening is to have a good morning meal to start the day off. And, likewise, the key to sleeping soundly and waking up feeling refreshed and ready to face the new day is to not go to sleep with undigested food in one's stomach.

It is for these reasons that I present before you what is known as the two-meal-a-day plan. It is one of the most important aspects for a successful diet and health plan, and I highly recommend you give it your full attention. Based upon everything presented here before, we know that we must eat enough food to satisfy our nutritional needs, but without interfering with any of the other essential body systems, such as sleep. It is far more important that we receive the correct quality of food, rather than focus on quantity. Our bodies can only handle so much food at a time.

If we overload our systems with excess food, it will lead to eventual breakdown by ingesting more nutrients than our bodies were designed to receive. Unfortunately, because our society has become so accustomed to overloading our bodies with great excess, we have come to accept this way of living as the "norm" as with so many other widely-accepted, but destructive, habits. Though I am not basing any of this book on scientific research, I thought it would be appropriate to mention here that the only 100 percent, absolutely proven way to extend the human lifespan is this: long-term calorie restriction.

When God took His people out of Egypt into the wilderness, He wanted to reintroduce them to the original diet He had given to our parents. So He gave them manna every day. There was a morning meal and an evening meal. He gave them the perfect eating schedule for eating the perfect food, and it was designed to ideally nourish them during their 40-year journey through the wilderness.

When we eat foods such as fresh fruits, leafy greens, nuts, and seeds, we are putting the most perfect, clean-burning food we can get on this earth into our bodies. Yet, it only does us good if it is eaten in the proper amount: not too much, not too little. The "more is always better" way of thinking that has so completely integrated itself into our society has led to a new form of gluttony. It is "health-food gluttony." We have been deceived by various nutritionists and healthcare practitioners that we are in danger of being deficient in all forms of nutrients. Therefore, they say that we must supplement our diets with an endless variety of potions and pills that they prescribe. This is truly a major deception, and it is totally based upon lack of faith.

Let us review the words of our Master: "Therefore take no thought, saying, What shall we eat? or, What shall we drink? or, Wherewithal shall we be clothed? (For after all these things do the Gentiles seek:) for your heavenly Father knoweth that ye have need of all these things. But seek ye first the kingdom of God, and his righteousness; and all these things shall be added unto you" (Matt. 6:31–33).

So, our Lord is telling us not to worry about all these "extras" as do the Gentiles, non-believers, for if we have faith, "all these things shall be added unto you." It is not by taking a new supplement or "superfood" or by drinking quantities of juice that we shall be nourished. Rather, we shall be nourished by finding a physical and spiritual balance with and through the Lord, and this is done by following all of His natural remedies, especially the one of trusting in God.

Why is the plan of eating twice a day and having nothing in between so important? Because it is crucial to establishing a sense of physical balance, which is equally essential to establishing balance with God and with our fellow humans. No matter what others have told you, your physical nature has a direct effect, in every way, with your spiritual nature. We are not "ghosts" temporarily residing in solid bodies! God created us as complete beings with a physical, mental, and spiritual nature. Our minds are not transient and separate from our physical bodies. Our very thoughts and memories consist of electronic and chemical reactions that take place within living brain cells. It is really a contradiction to say, "what affects the body affects the mind," for the mind is just a *part* of the body! The same blood that nourishes the liver and the skin also nourishes the brain. For these reasons, it is wise to make sure that one's bloodstream is kept as pure as possible.

Historical evidence shows that the ancient Hebrews traditionally ate only twice daily. This is really not unusual, as all throughout history, up to the present day, societies everywhere have subsisted upon only two meals a day. It really is the norm. The habit of dining heartily three times a day, not to mention snacking, are forms of gluttony shown in very prosperous societies such as our own. It is a custom that is the direct outgrowth of continually having more food (usually of a poor quality) than what is actually needed. Eating for "drunkenness" rather than "for strength" is directly tied to mainstream American culture. In this way, and in many others, we have truly become as the overindulgent ancient kingdom of Babylon.

Based upon all the above information, we can easily extrapolate an ideal schedule for mealtimes. After starting the day with a good, nourishing breakfast, about six hours should be allowed for the body to both digest the food therein, as well as prepare for the reception of the next meal. That would obviously mean that if breakfast is eaten early in the morning, let's say about 7 a.m., then dinner, or the mid-day meal, should be early in the afternoon, perhaps about 1 p.m. or so, depending upon one's personal schedule. An evening meal should only be eaten if one's digestion and vital powers are so weak that one cannot adequately digest any substantial amount of food at one meal. And, if the third meal is eaten, it should be light, consisting of fruit or some light leafy greens, so as not to interfere with sleep.

True hunger does not consist of an empty, bottomless pit feeling in one's stomach, accompanied by growling and rumbling sensations. True hunger is actually a pleasant, peaceful sensation that is more centered around feelings of the palate, and not that of the stomach. Overeating is simply another form of food addiction that can and will be overcome if one stands firm.

One of the largest of all lies in the "more is better" nutritional philosophy is that we cannot adequately "assimilate" the nutrients from whole foods unless they are altered by being liquefied or having the fiber completely removed, leaving only water and nutrients. More often than not, these false natural theories are spread abroad by those desiring to sell expensive machines and are not based upon any actual truths.

Chewing is the first part of the entire digestive process, and is far more essential to the digestion, absorption, and metabolization of food than most are aware of. While the fiber of the food is being broken down in the chewing process, the stomach receives signals, not only that food is coming but what kind of food is coming, and prepares itself by secreting the appropriate juices and enzymes for digestion. Regularly consuming blended or juiced foods completely bypasses this essential element in our body's utilization of the food we eat. Blended foods should only be regularly consumed by those who are unable to chew their food because of dental problems, etc. Blending and juicing one's food before eating also encourages eating much larger quantities of food than would otherwise be consumed.

Juicing advocates and home-juicer salespersons often speak of the fiber in food as "holding back" the absorption of needed nutrients into the bloodstream, and therefore, the most healthy way to get these needed nutrients is to remove the fiber and drink the juice, preferably through the means of a juicer that they are trying to sell you. This false statement is a result of people everywhere looking for another "quick fix" for their health without having to make any major changes in their own lifestyle habits.

If people would follow the laws of health that God gave us, we wouldn't need any "quick fixes." One of the notable dangers of this "juice-gluttony" is that by removing the fiber more nutrients are literally being dumped into the bloodstream than it is prepared to handle. This may have an exhilarating effect, a "rush" if you will, but it is not at all healthy, as the body now must work overtime to deal with this unnecessary excess of nutrients in the blood. The result is that the vast majority of nutrients are excreted from the body without ever actually reaching the cells of the body.

Fiber, when properly chewed, never "holds back" the absorption of any essential nutrients from the bloodstream. In fact, it actually regulates the absorption of the nutrients throughout the entire gastrointestinal tract so that it may be properly digested and then utilized by the body. Without the regulatory effect of fiber in our foods, digestion and nutrient absorption literally goes haywire! All nutrients that the human body needs, including fats and oils, are found in the natural, whole foods that God gave at Creation, and we should always acknowledge that God's ideals are the ideal! No exceptions. We do not have to take supplements or consume animal products to get our essential fats. Nuts, seeds, and avocados are some of the most delicious and enjoyable foods found in nature. They were made for us to consume. These natural fats and oils are completely digestible, whereas it has been said that a single tablespoon of oil taken with a meal can delay digestion for hours.

Let's examine some of the words of Paul regarding the body of Christ, that is, the church. Though he speaks of God's church, I think it could be looked upon as a parable to our food. You see, all of God's creation should be respected just as He made it in its whole, natural state. We need all the parts of God's original diet for humanity in order for our bodies to work properly.

Paul wrote, "For the body is not one member, but many. If the foot shall say, Because I am not the hand, I am not of the body; is it therefore not of the body? And if the ear shall say, Because I am not the eye, I am not of the body; is it therefore not of the body? If the whole body were an eye, where were the hearing? If the whole were hearing, where were the smelling? But now hath God set the members every one of them in the body, as it hath pleased him. And if they were all one member, which were the body? But now are they many members, yet but one body. And the eye cannot say unto the hand, I have no need of thee: nor again the head to the feet, I have no need of you. Nay, much more those members of the body, which seem to be more feeble, are necessary: And those members of the body, which we think to be less honourable, upon these we bestow more abundant honour; and our uncomely parts have more abundant comeliness. For our comely parts have no need: but God hath tempered the body together, having given more abundant honour to that part which lacked: That there should be no schism in the body; but that all members should have the same care one for another" (1 Cor. 12:14–25).

Thus we should regard all of God's creation, remembering that He created different parts and that together they make the whole.

Chapter Fourteen

THE SALT OF THE EARTH

We know that a reduction in caloric intake over the long-term results in the increase of one's lifespan. As we cease from ingesting large amounts of "fuel," our bodies begin to slow down, cool down, and become more efficient. This is why the quality of the food we eat from day to day is of so much more importance than the quantity. Efficiency is the key word regarding human nutrition; extra weight just slows us down.

And the "extra weight" I refer to here is not just the flab that so many carry around on their bodies. The average person is loaded down with a lifetime's accumulation of toxic substances that wear them out and slow them down, and often these internal poisons hardly even register on the scale. A young, lean, athletic person can be extremely toxic within and not even know it. Usually because of their youth, their bodies haven't started to feel the full effects of disregarding nature's laws. What is often considered to be the normal effects of aging is actually the old, lifelong bad habits just starting to catch up with them.

One of the best ways we can keep our internal mechanisms in tip-top condition is by periodic fasting. Although fasting doesn't have to be planned, a planned program of regular fasting is truly one of the best ways of extending one's life and remarkably increasing the quality of one's life!

When we have an issue in life, whether it be an illness, extreme emotional distress, or an unresolved matter with God, there is nothing better than fasting. Yes, they did a lot of fasting in the Bible, both for health and spiritual reasons, and they knew what they were doing. The whole point of fasting is not based on the idea that there is anything wrong with food or eating itself, but rather for the physical rest and clarity of mind that it brings.

During a fast, one should drink enough water to satisfy thirst, but not too much, and unless one is a practiced habitual faster, one should not engage in any heavy work but should be in a relaxing environment. Although it is a commonly used term among juicing promoters, there is no such thing as a juice-fast. Actually, a "juice-feast" would be a more accurate description, as juice is just food with the fiber removed.

Jesus speaks favorably of fasting, and He even gives us instructions on how to do it: "Moreover when ye fast, be not, as the hypocrites, of a sad countenance: for they disfigure their faces, that they may appear unto men to fast. Verily I say unto you, They have their reward. But thou, when thou fastest, anoint thine head, and wash thy face; That thou appear not unto men to fast, but unto thy Father which is in secret: and thy Father, which seeth in secret, shall reward thee openly" (Matt. 6:16–18). Because Jesus and His disciples fasted this way, disregarding the sackcloth and ashes way of fasting often described in the Bible and practiced by the Pharisees, others did not realize if and when Jesus and His followers were even fasting at all. "Then came to him the disciples of John, saying, Why do we and the Pharisees fast oft, but thy disciples fast not? And Jesus said unto them, Can the children of the bridechamber mourn, as long as the bridegroom is with them? but the days will come, when the bridegroom shall be taken from them, and then shall they fast" (Matt. 9:14, 15).

We are now in that period of time that Jesus spoke of. He is the Bridegroom, and He has been taken from us bodily until His second coming, and now is the time when we are to fast. Now is not to be a time of feasting and revelry. The antediluvians made that mistake, as "they were eating and drinking, marrying and giving in marriage ... And knew not until the flood came, and took them all away; so shall also the coming of the Son of man be" (Matt. 24:38, 39).

"I fast twice in the week" (Luke 18:12). Even though this text was written in a parable where Jesus spoke critically of a certain Pharisee, it was not the fasting, but the Pharisee's pride in himself that Jesus was criticizing. The Pharisees were very well-educated men, being the sect among the Jews who were recognized as the rabbis, the teachers of Israel. The Pharisees regularly fasted—its health-promoting benefits were well-known then as they are now. But Jesus pointed out that the problem with the Pharisees fasting was the same root problem as with their public prayers and public displays when they gave their tithes and offerings. Their downfall was their pride in themselves and in the act. This is why Jesus told them, "But thou, when thou fastest ... appear not unto men to fast ... and thy Father, which seeth in secret, shall reward thee openly" (Matt. 6:17, 18).

Fasting once or twice every week is an incredibly health-promoting practice, although when first starting out, it may require a little getting used to. If once a week seems like too much, then go for once every two weeks, or even once a month. There are no absolutes. Just give it a try. Also, when one feels as if they need a "break" from eating, but don't want to completely fast, going on an all-fruit diet for one, two, or three days at a time is a wonderful way to "clean out the cobwebs" from the body and the mind once in a while. This is especially good for heavy thinkers who don't want to feel weighed down by their food when they need all their mental powers to be at top efficiency.

Inevitably, when the subject of fasting in the Bible is discussed, the question of the forty-day fasts done by Moses, Elijah, and Jesus is brought up. First, let me state that a lengthy fast of six weeks or more, taking in nothing more than water alone, is not a miracle. It is well documented that people all over the world and throughout history have performed such fasts, for both spiritual and for health reasons, and sometimes, I suppose, just to prove a point.

One of the biggest disadvantages of long fasts is it can lead one into a "binge and purge" mentality. Some people live an indulgent lifestyle and then fast to "cleanse" themselves when it would be far better to live a stable way of life following God's plan. For obvious reasons, living a Christian life of moderation in all things is a much better way to go. Let us remember the following text from Paul to the Corinthians:

"Whether therefore ye eat, or drink, or whatsoever ye do, do all to the glory of God" (1 Cor. 10:31).

As you look for ways to improve your diet, it may be difficult to find fresh fruits and vegetables during certain seasons. To deal with this, I recommend two things. First, invest in a low-temperature food dehydrator. This allows you to be able to dry and store fresh foods without removing the life force within them. Secondly, try experimenting with sprouting seeds. It can be a wonderful "indoor garden" that can not only nicely supplement a healthy diet, but can even take the place of fresh vegetables when supplies are low. It is very simple and basic to get started sprouting. All you need is a dish drain, some wide-mouth Mason jars, some cheesecloth, rubber bands, and finally, some seeds for sprouting, and you're all set to go. It is literally gardening without getting your hands dirty, and the results are always pleasing.

It's also worth mentioning here that another good investment for the home is to get one's own water distiller. This is particularly true if one is living in an area where fresh water supplies are difficult to obtain. If you want to stop buying commercial bottled water, but you want to have fresh, clean water readily available, you should purchase a distiller.

Another commonly asked question among the masses is that of whether we need to be concerned about how we combine our foods. There are a lot of theories on this subject, some of which have become quite widespread in recent times, but I have to say that the negatives of these various food-combining theories far outweigh any perceived positives. Why? First, food combining is not a product of natural law, and it does not promote eating naturally. It is designed to lead the self-indulgent on a perceived plan of living that will somehow "lift up" their level of health while they are eating in total violation of the laws of nature. Nothing can truly do that. It is one of many commercially motivated deceptions that are out there in order to popularize messages that are being taught to sell books. Also, food-combining can lead some into a great deal of anxiety about whether what they are eating are "properly combined" foods or not.

Eating simple meals consisting of the natural products of the earth, with the spirit of thanksgiving, is always the best formula for good digestion. Negative emotions and worrying can definitely lead to indigestion!

With all that said, nature does place its foods into basic classes that we should understand. They are as such:

1) positive, 2) negative, and 3) neutral. The positive foods are basically the sweet fruits. This is because both the fruits themselves and the fruit sugar they contain are the final end product of the plant combining the energy of the sun and the minerals of the earth together. These are the foods that God had told Adam in the garden "thou mayest freely eat." Fruits truly are the expression of life in that they were made specifically for food, consisting of the minerals of the earth (the "dust of the ground") and the energy of the sun (the "breath of life").

The negative foods are the opposite of sweet fruits in that they are the "receivers" of the elements of life, whereas fruits express those same elements. The negative foods include all the vegetables. Leafy greens, through the chlorophyll that gives them their green color, perform the amazing process of photosynthesis, by which the energy of the sun itself is received and made available for the rest of the plant. Roots also receive the nutrients directly from the soil, so that the rest of the plant may utilize it. Other parts of the plant other than the leaves and roots, such as the stems and shoots, are classed as negative foods, as they are involved with the processing of the sun energy from the leaves and the soil nutrients from the roots, so they can be used for the formation of fruits and seeds.

Because of the opposite nature of positive and negative foods, they should not be eaten together at the same meal. (It could even be said that sweet fruits are "sun" foods and vegetables are "moon" foods, and that eating them together causes a digestive "eclipse.")

Neutral foods can be eaten with both positive and negative foods. They include the non-sweet fruits, such as cucumbers and tomatoes, fatty fruits such as avocados, and sour fruits such as lemons and limes. Nuts and seeds are also neutral. Sprouts, unless eaten in a very early state of growth, should generally be classed as vegetables (and only seeds that are edible when unsprouted can be eaten very young).

What about salt? Should it be totally eliminated, or can it be used in moderation? Well, salt has gotten much of a "bad rap" over the years, but this is primarily because of the fact that nearly everybody in the western world suffers from salt poisoning! Salt, when overused, can be very destructive to health, but, like all things in life, it must simply be used in moderation. The trouble is that it's hard to be "moderate" about salt consumption when nearly everything one eats is filled with salt. Canned and frozen items, restaurant food, junk food, and fast food especially, contain a ton of excess salt. Unless everything you eat is made from scratch, you are most likely eating way more salt than what is healthy. So how much salt is healthy? Well, it helps to know first the symptoms of salt poisoning. Dehydration and an insatiable thirst. Bloating and water retention. Recurring headaches and aches and pains throughout the body. No, these things are not "normal" for a healthy person, and they are among the most common symptoms of excess salt consumption.

On the other hand, salt has a place in our regular daily diet plan. Rather than being deleterious to the health, it is actually essential for the blood. A little salt added to food is an important part of our health regime. I recommend getting the purest salt possible, such as sea salt or rock salt, that is free of additives.

I'd like to quote a couple of verses from Scripture regarding salt and its comparison to the Christian life. "Salt is good ... Have salt in yourselves, and have peace one with another" (Mark 9:50). "Let your speech be always with grace, seasoned with salt, that ye may know how ye ought to answer every man" (Col. 4:6). "Ye are the salt of the earth..." (Matt. 5:13).

Chapter Fifteen
BABYLON'S WORLDWIDE DECEPTION

In the book of Daniel, the name Babylon makes direct reference to the ancient kingdom that ruled during Daniel's own lifetime, whereas, the book of Revelation, when speaking of Babylon, refers symbolically to a power that will exercise great power and worldwide authority, persecute God's people, and deceive all the nations of the world just before Christ's coming. John describes Babylon in Revelation: "So he carried me away in the spirit into the wilderness: and I saw a woman sit upon a scarlet coloured beast, full of names of blasphemy, having seven heads and ten horns. And the woman was arrayed in purple and scarlet colour, and decked with gold and precious stones and pearls, having a golden cup in her hand full of abominations and filthiness of her fornication: And upon her forehead was a name written, MYSTERY, BABYLON THE GREAT, THE MOTHER OF HARLOTS AND ABOMINATIONS OF THE EARTH. And I saw the woman drunken with the blood of the saints, and with the blood of the martyrs of Jesus " (Rev. 17:3–6).

So, just who is this "whore of Babylon"? We know she is a great religious power, one with equally great political authority. A woman in prophecy, as the Bible shows us, is a church. A pure, holy woman, as shown in Revelation 12, is the true church of Christ, whereas a whore, as in Babylon, represents a false church that is ruled by Satan. So just how will this false religious power, this adulterous whore, actually go about to deceive the entire planet? "Thus with violence shall that great city Babylon be thrown down, and shall be found no more at all ... for by thy sorceries were all nations deceived" (Rev. 18:21, 23).

It says here that it is through sorcery that Babylon will go and deceive the world. Sorcery? Isn't that just male witches in dark rooms mixing potions and casting spells? What could be so deceptive about that? Wouldn't it take more than that to deceive the entire world? Yes, this is absolutely true, and this is why we must delve a little deeper into Scripture to find out what Satan's plan is for deceiving the world in the very last days.

When God begins a time of revival and reformation among His people, He brings them back to their roots—the Word of God and the beginning of Creation. Satan, on the other hand, tries to counter and cover these things through lies and deception, clouding the minds and blinding the eyes of everyone. God uses true healing to reach the hearts and souls of people. The devil, our enraged adversary, tries to destroy the health of our bodies, our mind, and our spirit, all the while using the ultimate deception, convincing us that we are being "healed" while he is actually bringing us closer to death!

God has a message of health and healing for this new era we are living in. It began in the modern age in America in the early nineteen century, and it continues on to this day. Satan's message of false healing has its roots buried deep in the ideas that no matter how you live, you are going to get sick, so you might as well accept it. And since disease is inevitable, the best way to deal with it is by using poisonous substances to suppress the disease symptoms, as well as other invasive, destructive methods of "treatment."

This "great system" of False healing thrives and profits by its deception and outright abuse of its followers, and it also possesses great political power worldwide. No one questions its great international authority, which is virtually immune to political control.

Modern sorcery is what we need to beware of in these troublous times, not so much ancient witchcraft, even though modern sorcery does have its roots in the ancient black arts. But now they are far more powerful and destructive than anything in past times. We know from Scripture that the whore of Babylon uses modern sorcery to deceive all the nations of the world in the last days.

So what else does Revelation say about this hellish black art? "Neither repented they of their murders, nor of their sorceries, nor of their fornication, nor of their thefts" (Rev. 9:21). "But the fearful, and unbelieving, and the abominable, and murderers, and whoremongers, and sorcerers, and idolaters, and all liars, shall have their part in the lake which burneth with fire and brimstone: which is the second death" (Rev. 21:8). "Blessed are they that do his commandments, that they may have right to the tree of life, and may enter in through the gates into the city. For without are dogs, and sorcerers, and whoremongers, and murderers, and idolaters, and whosoever loveth and maketh a lie" (Rev. 22:14, 15).

Suffice it to say that Scripture classifies sorcery along with the most heinous of sins, and anyone who practices it will certainly not be found in God's kingdom. However, the words "sorcerers" or "sorceries," as translated into English, do not really give the best definition for the words. To see the true meaning of these words, we need to turn to the original Greek that the Bible was written in. The ancient Greek words are the following: *pharmakeia*, which means medication or magic, and also the words *pharmakeus, pharmakon*, and *pharmakos*, which mean drug, potion, druggist, poisoner, and magician. It is from these ancient words that we have such words as pharmacy and pharmaceutical in English, and the meanings haven't changed! We pay homage to this ancient black art every time we go to the drug store and get our prescriptions filled.

Are you following the laws of God as written by His hand in Mother Nature, or are you supporting the giant, Babylonian-based mechanism for deceiving the world, known as sorcery? Make your choice now, as time is running out. Actually, the drugs and pharmaceuticals of today are based upon the same principles as that of the potions that ancient sorcerers prescribed. Disease symptoms are the body's attempt to heal itself, and it takes vital force and strength to accomplish that. By introducing poisonous substances into the body, the vital force is weakened; therefore, the symptoms are suppressed. Patients are thereby deceived into believing they are healed, when in actuality, they are sicker! Then, as the patient continues to take the pills and the potions to relieve their symptoms, dependencies and addictions develop, which the "health-practitioner" is more than happy to provide for! "Come on down, and I'll fix you right up!"

This is how the devil works, and how he always will work.

"Gall and wormwood," otherwise known as "poisonous herbs" (Deut. 29:18) are examples of the old potions used in the past, and though derived from nature, they were still highly toxic. The difference today is that everything is created with advanced technology, with new, even more poisonous substances than are normally found in nature, distilled down to their purest state for "maximum results."

It needs to be pointed out that drugs themselves are not evil. It is only when they are wrongly used that they became tools of evil. While Satan uses drugs widely in his worldwide system of false healing, we should consider the situation of the sheep in the pit, as Jesus spoke of it: "Is it lawful to heal on the sabbath days?... And he said unto them, What man shall there be among you, that shall have one sheep, and if it fall into a pit on the sabbath day, will he not lay hold on it, and lift it out? How much then is a man better than a sheep? Wherefore it is lawful to do well on the sabbath days" (Matt. 12:10–12). To revive a man having a heart attack, using a pharmaceutical agent, is definitely an example of what Christ is talking about here. Sorcery involves deception. Using a drug in a life-threatening emergency involves no deception at all. Regarding these matters, we must be as "wise as serpents, and harmless as doves" (Matt. 10:16). Always ask for God's guidance.

So-called "holistic healing" involves some of the greatest deceptions of all. It is definitely just another part of the great worldwide false healing movement that the devil is promoting today. Even though the "cures" may not be near as harmful as the treatments used by the established power of false healing, the idea is the very same: "When you get sick, come to me, and I'll heal you!" Although many of these systems of healing may seem natural and relatively benign, they are not only built upon false pretenses but many are founded upon ancient, heathen philosophies and ideas. The claim by some that they can "balance your energy" by sticking needles in your skin is not based upon any of God's laws of health and healing.

Even good things can be misused, as well. Massage can be very therapeutic because of the power in the human touch, but that is all. Virtually all of what is called herbal medicine or herbalism is based upon superstitious nonsense going back to times when plants were attributed to have healing properties within them, which they do not possess. No product of nature or anything else in creation has the ability to cure disease. All of the non-nutritional plants used in herbalism, both ancient and modern, have toxic, pharmaceutical effects that suppress symptoms, but that is it.

I am not addressing in detail right now the simple, natural remedies that temporarily help the body during times of sickness or weakness, such as poultices and hydrotherapy. But even these simple means require wisdom and discretion, as Satan would always like us to turn to remedies, even the good ones, rather than follow God's laws of health in our daily lives. People like to think that their illnesses, which so frequently afflict them, are just a matter of "chance," which, as Christians, we do not believe exists. They think that they just happened to be at the wrong place at the wrong time, or whatever, and that is why they are sick. Modern sorcery preys upon this denial and ignorance, as it simply feeds the idea that there is really nothing you can do, so why try?

One of the biggest and most deceptive lies that has virtually taken hold of nearly everyone as a result of sorcery's deceptions is the idea that microorganisms, germs, are one of the primary causes of all disease. "Germ paranoia" is running rampant. People think that by carefully sanitizing their hands every time they might touch something "unclean" they are taking a big step in avoiding disease! Well, guess what? Germs are everywhere, and they have a place in the great ecosystem. They cannot be avoided. Germs never prey upon and devour healthy flesh. They only consume sick, half-dead flesh.

Remember, "you are what you eat," and "a house is only as strong as the materials it is built with." Well, if our bodies are built with dead food, we will literally be "walking carcasses." Christ said, "For wheresoever the carcase is, there will the eagles be gathered together" (Matt. 24:28). If our bodies become a "germ motel," it is only because we have built them that way. Israel only became prey for the nation who had wings "as swift as the eagle flieth" when they didn't respect His laws and commandments. So shall it be for us in this day.

Our obsession with external cleanliness is a direct result of the filthiness and corruption we have kept stored up inside of our bodies for a lifetime. And in a vain attempt to remove some of the uncleanness, which we know permeates our very beings, we try to cleanse and scrub our bodies. We deodorize ourselves from putrid and foul smells that only naturally result from deep-buried toxins within our flesh. Some even become obsessed with keeping their material possessions, their houses and cars, "sparkling clean" to somehow offset in their minds the uncleanness that lie within themselves. But it is all foolishness and denial.

Anything short of getting to the very heart of the issue will never bring the results for which we are seeking—true health. The words of Christ to the Pharisees shed light on the matter: "Woe unto you, scribes and Pharisees, hypocrites! For ye make clean the outside of the cup and of the platter, but within they are full of extortion and excess. Thou blind Pharisee, cleanse first that which is within the cup and platter, that the outside of them may be clean also. Woe unto you, scribes and Pharisees, hypocrites! For ye are like unto whited sepulchres, which indeed appear beautiful outward, but are within full of dead men's bones, and of all uncleanness" (Matt. 23:25–27)

Babylon is using her sorceries right now to deceive the nations. It is predicted. It will happen. It is happening. Right now we need to take the mighty hand of our Great Physician, Jesus Christ, that we, His people, the body of Christ, may reach out to the world with our *Right Arm*—the message of health and healing for the soul—and thus show everyone the path that leads to truth and light.

RECOMMENDED READING

Confessions of a Medical Heretic by Robert S. Mendelsohn, M.D.

Country Living by Ellen G. White

Diet For A New America by John Robbins

The Great Controversy by Ellen G. White

In The Beginning, God Said: Eat Raw Food by William D. Scott

The Ministry of Healing by Ellen G. White

Raw Food Treatment of Cancer by Kristine Nolfi, M.D.

The Two-Meal-a-Day Plan by Laymen Ministries

We invite you to view the complete
selection of titles we publish at:

www.TEACHServices.com

Please write or email us your praises, reactions, or
thoughts about this or any other book we publish at:

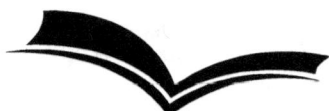

TEACH Services, Inc.
P U B L I S H I N G
www.TEACHServices.com • (800) 367-1844

P.O. Box 954
Ringgold, GA 30736
info@TEACHServices.com

TEACH Services, Inc., titles may be purchased in bulk
for educational, business, fund-raising,
or sales promotional use.
For information, please e-mail:

BulkSales@TEACHServices.com

Finally, if you are interested in seeing
your own book in print, please contact us at

publishing@TEACHServices.com

We would be happy to review your manuscript for free.